SEDUCED BY A RIVER

ADVENTURES IN LOVE, SEX, AND WHITEWATER

C.C. HAVENS

UTE PASS PRESS

Excerpt from DELTA OF VENUS: Erotica by Anais Nin. Copyright 1969 by Anais Nin. Copyright 1977 by The Anais Nin Trust. Used by permission of Houghton Mifflin Harcourt Publishing Company. All rights reserved.

Excerpt from Angels Would Fall by Melissa Etheridge used with permission.

PRINT ISBN 978-0-692-12659-2
Library of Congress Control Number: 2016931084

"…a wound of ecstasy and pleasure which rent her body like lightning, and let her fall again, moaning, a victim of too great a joy, a joy that was like a little death, a dazzling little death that no drug or alcohol could give, that nothing else could give but two bodies in love with each other, in love deep within their beings, with every atom and cell and nerve, and thought."
~ ANAIS NIN, *DELTA OF VENUS*

I've crept into your temple
I have slept upon your pew
I've dreamt of the divinity
Inside and out of you
I want it more than truth
I can taste it on my breath
I would give my life just for a little death

FROM: *ANGELS WOULD FALL* BY MELISSA ETHERIDGE

TABLE OF CONTENTS

FOREWORD

IN 2001, I was with the wrong man for all the right reasons. He was a nice guy. He loved my dog. He made me laugh.

But the passion and emotional commitment that was lacking in our relationship made me cry as well. I was lonely in love.

After seven years, we'd never followed through on the engagement and we were no longer living together. But neither one of us could quite let go.

"You two are so stuck," said my college girlfriend Marie.

I knew she was right but I didn't know what to do about it. An imperfect lover was better than no lover at all. I was playing it safe.

The previous year I had completed a yoga teacher training at the Kripalu Center for Yoga and Health, so I sought solace on my mat and meditation cushion. One word kept rising to the surface of my stormy thoughts like a life raft:

Trust.

I floated upon it for months and let go of my obsession of trying to figure things out. I shifted my focus away from the circuitous way I had been trying to get love—by showering it on my boyfriend thinking that it would run off of him and back to me—which it didn't. Instead, I started mainlining pranyama and the loving kindness metta. I found myself channeling all my romantic longing and sexual fantasies into an erotic romance novel. My female protagonist had not one, but two sexy men of the American West vying for her attention. A year into the draft of that story, a man walked into my yoga studio who was a mind-blowing montage of both my male leads blended into one.

"Oh my God, you manifested him," said my writing buddy Mical who'd read every chapter of my novel.

My prince didn't ride in on a white horse. He showed up in a red Nissan truck with two kayaks, a raft, a mountain bike, a road bike and a pair of skis strapped to the top, an adventurer right out of the pages of the Patagonia catalogue. He meditated, practiced yoga and was the most open-hearted, passionate man I'd ever met, an embodiment of this mountain yogini's greatest fantasy.

I lay awake at night thinking about the sexy outdoor guide who was now trading me elk meat for yoga classes.

"Follow the energy," said my older sister Susie.

It was the best advice I've ever taken. I quit playing it safe. Before I could say *Om Shanti* I was snowmobiling in to his remote cabin in the snowy Rockies; backcountry skiing in the Tetons; paddling Class IV + rivers and backpacking through the rugged bush of New Zealand.

To top it all off, unlike my previous long-term, non-committed boyfriends, this man wanted to marry me. While trail-running on New Zealand's Kaikoura Peninsula, he tackled me in the wildflowers and proposed.

As you can imagine (you won't have to for long if you keep reading) the sex was... I don't want to steal my own thunder here so I'll just point out the obvious: the sex inspired me to abandon the fictional characters of my novel (I still feel kind of bad about that) and start writing an erotic memoir.

I kept pinching myself, wondering when I was going to wake up, and then I did, ten months into my marriage when I recognized a huge oversight on my part. I wasn't the only object of my passionate man's passion. I had some formidable competition in the *femme-fatale* essence of white water who seduced him away from me for months at a time.

I found myself alone in love.

I did yoga and meditated *a lot, again,* because I obviously had more to learn and besides, he left me with his off-the-grid cabin on 120 acres (a retreat center if there ever was one) with all my abandonment and rejection issues rearing their ugly, needy heads. I ended up at my keyboard over and over, determined to understand the threesome dynamics of my marriage.

And what I eventually came up with was this:

I could stay home alone and worry about the river taking him from me forever or I could tag along and risk dying myself.

So I went.

I found myself in over my head in some of the most beautiful and remote rivers and mountains in the American West and in the process, tapped into some pretty wild states of ecstasy. Hanging out on that razor sharp edge of adventure is physically, emotionally and spiritually intense, but I kept going back for more because fear is an oddly powerful aphrodisiac and the *femme-fatale* expression of the divine femininity of nature is incredibly, organically erotic.

My man's lust for whitewater and adventure, his mistress, became my nemesis and my muse and writing about her has not only kept me sane but it has kept the passion alive in my marriage. Thirty-six essays and many adventures later, I'd like to think that I've figured out a few things that you might find thought-provoking, arousing or at the very least, sensual and fun to read.

So my story starts where most fairy tales and romance novels end. My story starts when I crawled to my meditation cushion, determined to keep a very tight and unspiritual grip on my Happily Ever After. My story starts when in a moment of desperation, I cut a deal with the river. All these years later, I'm still trying to hold up my end of the bargain.

These essays were written as gifts to my husband and ended up fueling my determination to have a sexy, passionate, long-term relationship. My hope is that they will inspire your love relationship or your vision of one.

Because we all deserve a Happily Ever After.

May these pages lead you toward a deeper exploration of your beautifully complicated erotic self, much as writing them did for me.

Enjoy,
C.C. Havens

PROLOGUE

May 2008

I'M GETTING SPANKED. By a queen.

Oh, how I wish she was a gorgeous drag queen, laughing in her husky voice as she punishes me for sneaking into her blue glitter mascara. Or better yet, Cate Blanchett dressed in full queen regalia slapping my reddening buttocks with her delicate white-skinned hand. But right now, I'd gladly offer up my bare bum to stern old Elizabeth armed with a royal wooden paddle.

Anything, really, but this.

Because I disrespected a wild and unpredictable queen, the queen of all river trips, the 297-mile stretch of the Colorado River that runs through the Grand Canyon. And when this queen decided to teach me a lesson, she started spanking so hard she's taking my breath away. As my body tumbles and churns beneath the aqua-colored water of one of her more formidable rapids, I am starting to wonder if she's ever going to give it back.

I've heard that in those final moments before death, your entire life flashes in front of your eyes. For me, it's the last three and a half years, undoubtedly the most erotic of my forty-two. I know it's strange to be thinking about orgasms, what the French refer to as *la petite mort*, 'the little deaths', when I am quite possibly facing a big, white watery one. But if I'm going down, and I am indeed getting pulled deeper into this violent hydraulic, it only makes sense that I'd be thinking about my husband, the man who was on the oars of this raft that flipped on top of me, the man who has brought me to the kind of transcendent states of sexual ecstasy that I spent my twenties and early thirties fantasizing about. It's probably best to have my last thoughts be of sex with my man than this queen bitch of a river that is trying to seep between my lips, but then again, who am I trying to kid? The two have never been mutually exclusive. When I fell head over heels (hiking boots actually) and married a raft guide, the river was a non-negotiable part of the package.

And as you can see, our threesome relationship… it gets a little intense sometimes.

CHAPTER ONE

August 2005
Possession

MY HUSBAND IS WITH HIS MISTRESS.
She summons him on the first soft breeze of spring and he goes without a backward glance, eager for the plunge. For six weeks, she lures him West from our home in Colorado to the California Salmon River, seducing his kayaker's soul with her warm, green-water rapids. He doesn't come home until *she* is ready: when the Arkansas and Colorado Rivers run white in mid- July.

I try not to compete; I have no choice but to share.

But not tonight.

Tonight, I have convinced my husband of ten months to join me at our secluded cabin in the mountains, away from his river and all her whitewater turbulence I have yet to understand. After weeks of feeling like a fledgling guppy as I attempted to learn his sport, I yearn to be on solid ground. I want to breathe in the musk of his arousal intertwined with the scent of sage that wafts in our bedroom window.

I sip white wine and watch the mango-and-plum-colored sunset. I feel juicy tonight, like the sky, the flesh of my sex warm and moist against the worn denim of my cut-offs. My kayaker will be here any minute, and I can hardly wait to reclaim him. His dark hair will be tousled from the river's winds, his torso bronzed and chiseled from navigating her rapids all week. I'm so excited I can hardly sit still. So I don't. I lower the stem of my wine glass between my thighs and push myself against its hardness.

I am as wet as a river.

*   *   *

The fruit-salad sunset is long gone and my lover has yet to arrive. I sit in the dark and sip hot tea, listening to the cries of a lone coyote. Despite the warmth of the summer night, I am chilled to the bone. I've done the math a hundred different times on how many hours it should take for his afternoon kayak run and drive across the mountains. By ten thirty, the numbers quit adding up. I feel growing tendrils of worry, wondering if he went out on the river alone. Not many of his co-workers are as passionate about the river as he is. After a day of guiding clients down the river, they are ready to kick back with a cold beer. Would he take the risk, defy safety and kayak solo to get in one last run?

I know he would.

I remind myself that he's been paddling that stretch of the Arkansas River for sixteen years. He knows her every bend and curve even better than he knows mine, but by eleven thirty, the worry has grown in me like an aggressive cancer. Just last week, a kayaker died on the nearby Poudre River when he was pinned under water by a powerful current.

I wonder if the river, like me, is tired of sharing him. I imagine her taking advantage of this rare opportunity to have him all alone, pulling him into her depths and holding him there, much like I wanted to do this weekend.

I pull my knees to my chest beneath his large, fleece jacket and look up at the stars shimmering overhead like spilled glitter. Our cabin is off-the-grid on 120 acres, a twenty-minute drive to the nearest neighbor. Although this affords us one of the rarest things, a dark night sky, it also deprives us of one of the most ordinary, cell phone coverage. I think back to our last phone conversation when I suggested this cabin rendezvous. He didn't want to leave the river. I didn't want to meet him there again.

For the past two months, I've been dipping my toes in her waters, trying to make friends. And I think she likes me. I haven't been sucked into a hydraulic hole or pummeled in a rapid…yet. But from the stories I hear from all our river friends, it is just a matter of time. I remember the words of our friend Dave, my kayak instructor on the Salmon River. "The river is so forgiving...until she's not."

I'm tired of wondering when she is going to quit being so forgiving, tired of being upside down in a boat that I can't always roll back over. But I am even more fed up with the grip she has on my husband. He should be here with me in our cabin, drinking wine and making passionate love. Instead, he had to be with her one more time.

I feel so pathetic: I'm jealous of a body of water. But what a body. She's wild and wet and has curves that just don't stop. She's beautiful and dangerous, the ultimate femme fatale. If plunging in a phallus-shaped boat into a tight, gushing gorge isn't sexual, what is?

I told him he was obsessed.

He couldn't deny it. He tried to explain his passion for the river, his dark brows furrowing as he struggled to find an analogy I would understand. "Kayaking is just another way to hook in...like yoga...or meditation. I have to be so present and focused that nothing else exists but me and the river. And then, it's just the river."

He wants so much to share it with me. I want so much to experience it. After eight weeks of trying, I am nowhere close.

Time inches toward midnight. I move my vigil into the cabin and grab a dharma book from the bookshelf, seeking solace in Buddhist philosophy. My meditation practice has been a good friend this summer, reminding me to be present, to stay calm under water, to name fear. I need a friend right now.

But the dharma is fucking with me tonight. The words that come off the page lend no comfort. Attachment. Grasping. And the one that makes my eyes burn with tears. Impermanence.

I toss the book aside and grab my meditation cushion, deciding that I will sit until midnight and then, if he still isn't here, I'll drive out until I can pick up cell coverage. I focus on my breath, naming the worry, the jealousy, the fear. I recognize the irony that I planned this weekend to take a break from all my confusing emotions around the river, and here I sit consumed by them.

Alone in the dark with my churning thoughts, I find myself reaching out to the river. I beg her not to be as selfish as me, beg her not to take the beautiful man it took me thirty-seven years to find.

I speak to her in the darkness: *I'll share. I'll share. I'll share.*

Instantly I hear the faint groan of his truck as it navigates our rugged two-track driveway. As the sound grows louder, I buckle forward, whispering a silent prayer of gratitude that he is safe. I thank the river for not taking him.

A wave of relief washes over me and I am surprised by the undertow of emotion that follows. Now that I know he is alive and safe, I want to kill him. Anger is so much easier than raw vulnerability.

I stand as he steps into the cabin. He sees my tears and pulls me tight into the hardness of his chest and apologizes for being so late. Not wanting to paddle alone, he convinced several of his co-workers to join him on the river and consequently everything took three times as long. He knew I'd be worried. He is so sorry he couldn't call. I'm too tired to talk and know better than to try when I feel like this. We crawl up the stairs to our bedroom loft, tender and tired. We lie naked together, curl up like worn pups, and sleep.

*   *   *

In the dark hours of morning, the river awakens me with a whisper.

Feel my current...

A light caress drifts across my belly. I recognize the calloused hand as my husband's, but the delicate, fluid touch is unfamiliar. His hand floats up and down my body like a wave, tracing the curves of my hip, the swell of my breast, the arousal of my nipple. By the slow cadence of his breathing I can tell he is sleeping, touching me from his dreams. As I roll to my side, his body follows, spooning around me. He mutters something unintelligible; under the silence that follows I hear her again.

Feel my flow...

Gently, she urges his hips into the back of mine, swaying our bodies in unison as his hand presses against my sex. Light kisses drift across my shoulder and up my neck like a soft breeze. Reaching through the leaden layers of sleep toward this ecstasy, this seduction, I begin to understand. She is here. I recognize my husband's obsession for the river for what it truly is. Possession.

Feel my passion...

As she nuzzles my neck, the roughness of my husband's two-day beard sends a current down my body where his fingers swirl and explore my folds. Her kisses become more ardent as I let my head fall back, as my lips meet his.

Feel my wetness…

My parched lips are engulfed in the moistness of her, his tongue is soft and wet as it tangles with mine. His fingers are slick from my arousal, circling deeper and deeper until she finds my sweet spot with his thumb. And then, she dives. Kisses drip down my belly like warm rain. I feel the velvet of his tongue as she drinks me in, his hands tight on the flesh of my hips.

Feel my waves…

He begins to undulate my body, pulsing my sex against his face, his nose pushing against my clitoris while his tongue entices my entrance. She is moving, moving through me, a rapid of pure pleasure. I begin to quiver.

Feel my power…

His lips glisten as she rises, arching his back and expanding his chest above me like a king cobra. She slides his erection against my clitoris. She rocks against my slickness. She convulses me in waves.

I reach for her, eager to taste my orgasm on his lips and find myself mesmerized by the smooth, green stone that has hung from his neck since the day I met him. I reach for the dark jade that was harvested from the Salmon River, his river talisman, and kiss it.

Yes…Yes…

I move the stone into my mouth and suck, working the smooth hardness of it in and out across my lips. I can almost feel her shudder.

We'll share. We'll share. We'll share.

I suck her hard into the back of my throat. I guide my husband deep inside me.

I hold them there.

CHAPTER TWO

December 2005
Abstinence

I AM WET WITH DESIRE.

My mouth salivates at the sight of my man sitting beside me. It's not the sexy hint of silver at his temples or the hardness of his chest straining against his polypropylene T-shirt. I'm not craving his lips, his tongue or his cock.

I am lusting after his grilled cheese sandwich.

I swallow hard as he takes the first bite. As his teeth penetrate the thick sprouted-wheat bread, I hear the soft crunch of the buttery grilled crust. I squirm in my wood chair as the cheese stretches out from his lips. I imagine leaning over, sucking the strand of chewy mozzarella into my mouth and letting it seduce me back to all that bready bliss.

But I don't.

I scrape the last spoonful of my lentil brown rice soup into my mouth and try to distract myself with the bowl of fruit on the kitchen table. This tactic lasts about five seconds. My gaze gravitates back to his plate, lured by the heady aroma of warm buttery bread.

It's a classic case of the lure of the forbidden. Some women secretly lust after their best friend's teenage son. Others fantasize about seducing their married co-worker. For me, it's bread.

I haven't had wheat in three months. No chewy toasted bagels lathered in cream cheese. No dense pumpernickel warm out of the oven saturated with butter. Why?

After catching every cold that infiltrated my small mountain community the past two years, I decided to go on a mission to strengthen my immune system. Coincidentally, an old friend called the next day and spoke of his mother-in-law and her determination to fight cancer. A naturopathic doctor suggested that she quit eating refined sugar and wheat to strengthen her immune system after the devastation of chemotherapy. Like a good hypoglycemic, I'd already cut most of the sugar from my diet years ago and the idea of eliminating wheat sounded intriguing. I decided to try it.

Unfortunately, it worked. While my friends and yoga students suffer with various colds, flus and viruses, I've been immune. Not even a sniffle.

I can't quit now.

But my resolve is crumbling like a blueberry muffin. Abstinence isn't my forte. But neither is coughing up green phlegm. It's simply a choice. Well, maybe not that simple.

Right now I want those two pieces of golden brown bread wrapped around all that oozing cheese more than anything. We climbed over 4500 vertical feet on our telemark skis today. I deserve it. My dinner of soup and rye crackers is long gone and feels like air inside my belly.

My man's sandwich is almost a memory. He eats it fast, mechanically, as if it isn't the most amazing thing in the world. To him it is just fuel. If it was mine, I would chew slowly, savoring and cherishing it like a final kiss from a lover at the airport. I seriously consider reaching over and snatching the last bite.

But I don't.

I grab the apple from the bowl of fruit as he pops the last bit of crust into his mouth and licks his fingers. Feeling a pang of grief for my unfulfilled hedonistic self, I bite ravenously into the apple, a bite so big that the sweet juices overflow and dribble down my chin. My skier swallows and stares greedily at me.

"That looks good," he says as he leans forward, licks the juice from my chin, and reaches for my apple.

My hand snaps back. I am not sharing.

The apple is extended far behind me as our lips meet. I taste the earthy glutinous wheat, the thick oils of the butter and cheese on his lips. Suddenly, I want to devour him. I kiss and lick all around his lips. They taste slick, salty and reminiscent of yeast. My tongue dives deep into his mouth, hungry for more.

His arms, much longer than mine, get the apple. He licks the juices off the exposed, pale flesh and kisses me again. Our tongues dance, a tango of tastes: wheat, sweet, buttery, juicy. My tongue slides down his neck exploring the saltiness of his skin from our day of exertion. I grab the apple, rub it down his neck and lick slowly, from his collarbone to his ear, savoring every inch of his sweet, salty taste.

He takes the apple from me and tosses it on the table. He pulls my fleece sweater over my head, releasing my hair from its ponytail and then guides me towards the soft rug in front of the woodstove.

It's time for dessert. The sweetest kind.

CHAPTER THREE

January 2006
Mounting Hailey

I AM MOMENTARILY BLINDED by snow as Black Betty hits a dip in the trail and goes airborne. Sitting behind my man with a silly grin on my face, I am Hobbes to his Calvin as our snowmobile lands, leaving my stomach somewhere behind us on the trail. Our legs straddle the duct-taped vinyl seat, my pubis glued to his tailbone. As his body moves from side to side, mine follows, leaning and lunging to keep old Betty on the trail as we bust through a foot of fresh powder. We hit a straightaway and the engine whines as he opens up the throttle to gather speed. When I peek over his shoulder and see what's coming, my arms cinch tighter around his waist as I bury my face into his upper back.

Black Betty moans and nearly stalls as we plunge straight into a four-foot-high snow drift. When we come out on the other side, laughing and choking on snow, we pause for a high five and some goggle maintenance.

"Look at her." Even though my backcountry skier's voice is muffled beneath layers of fleece and Gortex, I can still detect an intonation of lust. I follow his gaze over aspen branches fuzzy with hoarfrost and hone in on the object of his affection.

Peaking at 11,000 feet and dominating our cabin's view to the south, Mount Hailey definitely meets mistress criteria. She's remote, gorgeous, physically challenging to mount, and dangerous. In the spring, her snow pack melts, transforming into white water. She is, in effect, a winter manifestation of the river, all vamped up in a fluffy white coat. And my adventurer gets just as obsessed with skiing her white powdery curves in the winter as he does kayaking her white watery ones in the summer.

It's been an unpredictable, passionate affair, this love between the remote mountain and the avid backcountry skier. The past few years have been wrought by painful separations, prompted first by drought and then by educational pursuits. When they did commune, it was random, spontaneous and usually just the two of them. This winter, with the phenomenal early season snow and a keen bride in tow, it's been a full-on threesome.

In one of my favorite photographs from our wedding ceremony, I am standing next to my groom in a full-length, sage-green lace dress that I found at a lingerie store. He is wearing dark green Carharts and a burlap and rust-colored shirt we splurged on from Ralph Lauren. Between our heads, in the background, stands Mount Hailey. It is so appropriate. I married that mountain too. As if knowing this, she dressed for the occasion. In the photo, her peak sparkles with the first September snow; her evergreen base dappled with the shimmering gold of autumnal aspen leaves.

Today she is pure white from head to toe looking both seductive and virginal all at the same time. I look up at her and feel two emotions churning in my belly. Fear, because she's been known to slide; and arousal because plunging down her untracked meadows, glades and chutes is nothing short of orgasmic. Skiing her is an all-day dance between the two.

Some lovers explore sadomasochism with handcuffs, whips and chains. We mount Hailey.

We travel the last mile to her base, park the snowmobile and begin to strip.

For the next hour or so we will be climbing non-stop uphill. We pare down to polypro, fleece and sunglasses and cram the Gortex jackets, knit hats and goggles into our ski packs. We clip on our avalanche beacons, secure our climbing skins to the bottom of our skis and start our approach. As my man navigates a short, downhill pitch through the pines at the beginning of the trail, I pause.

"Hey, Beauty," I whisper. I have to admit it has taken me a while to warm up to Hailey. Like the river, she's intimidating as hell. Even though I grew up on skis, the biggest threat on the ski slopes of Northern Michigan was frost bite. Hailey is a little different. If you try to ski her north face too early in the season, like my adventurer dared to do one year, you can get spanked. Or die. Hailey gave him just enough time to ski into the trees and then buried him up to his knees just to make sure he got the message. She didn't like it when we lingered too long on a sunny day last spring either. I've never been so happy to be off a mountain after she bombarded us with wet slides on our final descent.

She demands respect. I'm willing to give it.

I bow in reverence at the edge of the trees and recite my adventure mantra.

May we be safe.

When I first met my adventurer, I concluded that he was fearless. He skied avalanche chutes and paddled Class V whitewater. He launched heart first into our love affair and committed to a long-distance relationship after just eight amazing days and nights together. With time, I realized he wasn't immune to fear, he was just comfortable with it. He knew how to harness it, like a wild horse, and ride it. This was a new concept for me. I'd always instinctively moved away from scary, dangerous situations until he showed me how fun it was on that razor-sharp edge.

I'm slowly overcoming my fear of getting buried by one of Hailey's avalanches because skiing her is such an ultimate life experience. I justify the risk of dying, because what kind of life would I have, knowing this kind of ecstasy exists but not embracing it? Besides, if she takes me down, and this is a reality, I'm sure there are worse ways to die than being swallowed whole by a mountain.

I follow my skier's lead through lodgepole pines and stop as he traverses the base of one of her avalanche chutes. As I watch him, I mentally rehearse how calm I will be if she slides. I'll use my beacon to search for the signal emitted from his. I'll dismantle my poles and reassemble them into a probe to locate his buried body. I will dig as fast as I can without freaking. It's morbid, I know, but it is the reality of making love to a mountain on backcountry skis.

When my man is clear of the avalanche area, I ski in his tracks as he, now, watches me. When I am out of the danger zone, we fall into a kick-and-glide climbing rhythm as we begin our ascent.

Maybe I'm projecting, but I swear she gets excited when she sees us coming up out of the trees. I get the sense that she is just aching to be climbed and wants it as badly as we do. Like any fun lover, she makes us work for it.

The ascent, like foreplay, is half the pleasure. As we break trail up her east face, she is a blatant flirt, letting her wide-open, untracked snowfields sparkle at us under the early morning sun. When we pause to flip up our climbing bars, she flaunts the clean lines through her aspen stands, and teases us with her steep avalanche chutes that won't be stable enough to ski for another month. Her trees brush their branches against the top of our packs, urging us upward as we grunt and sweat our way up her winding 1500 feet of vertical that warms us no matter how cold the wind chill is. By the time we summit, our bloodstreams pulse with endorphins. We pull on Gortex shells, knit hats and goggles and peel off our climbing skins. Beneath our fleece our bodies are hard, wet and ready.

Knowing her as he does, my adventurer goes first, warming to the mood of the snow on her east face. This route is the safest descent, but there is one steep pitch that could slide, so as soon as he drops out of sight, I follow, spooning my turns right next to his tracks. As I lunge into my telemark turns, I feel her fluttering up between my thighs, a titillating percussive against my labia. I lunge deeper with the next turn and am rewarded with a cool kiss that melts quickly on my lips. I lick them, tasting her and stroke her back with the carve of my turn. She floats over my shoulder, caressing my back as I hug her contours with my skis. When her vertical incline increases, I scan the slope for any signs of an avalanche. I am relieved to see nothing but my man's serpentine ski tracks dropping steeply into a glade of pines.

I remind myself to stay forward on my skis despite the instinctual urge to lean back.

Lead with your heart, lead with your clit.

I push my chest straight down the fall line, keep my poles in front of me and for a moment I feel as if I am flying, no longer held by the earth, but buoyed by one of her most magical mediums, snow so dry and inebriating that it has been dubbed champagne powder. I make love, one turn at a time, to this mountain and she loves me right back, grazing my crotch, breasts and lips with her powdery caress. I giggle despite the fact that my third turn is totally lame and doesn't check my speed. I digress quickly from skiing with my clit to skiing with my ass on the tails of my skis, rendering me completely out of control. I bail and fall sideways into the mountain and slide to a stop right before I hit a pine tree where my skier stands waiting. I lie on my back, my arms flung open, a huge grin on my face.

"Nice!" He reaches down and brushes snow off my hat.

I love the sensation of being covered with her so I sit in the snow and try to catch my breath between bouts of uncontrollable laughter. I am thrilled that I finally got at least two good turns in on the east-side steeps.

"Oh. My. God." I get out between breaths. "That. Was. Amazing."

"You're getting it. You really nailed those first two turns." He is always the encourager, ignoring the fact that I blew the second two.

"That first turn...as I came into the steep pitch...I was so there...clit first and everything. And at the very top, those pussy flutters!"

"Pussy flutters?"

"Yeah, pussy flutters. You didn't get any?"

His left eyebrow lifts conveying: *I don't have a pussy.*

"I mean, testicle tickles. Crotch shots. She didn't give you any?"

"You are much shorter than me."

"Maybe you should try deeper turns."

"Maybe we can't afford knee surgery." He grabs my hand and pulls me up. He kisses my lips that are dusted with snow. I feel her melt between us.

"Maybe she just likes me more."

He ignores that possibility. "Pussy flutters, huh? Kind of like this?" He lowers his glove between my thighs and drums his fingers against the crotch of my ski pants.

"Yes," I say leaning into his touch, "a lot like that. Just a little wispier, like this." I reach over and flutter my fingers between his thighs.

"Skiing with an erotica writer sheds a whole new light on things."

He traverses through the pines and I follow until we reach the meadow that was blatantly flirting with us as we made our ascent. She's winking at us now, a thousand eyes sparkling in the sun. The angle of the slope is just under thirty degrees, so there is no threat of avalanche here. This is the kind of run that makes any skier wet: untracked, fresh snow on a wide-open slope that funnels into a stand of widely spaced aspen. But there are never any other skiers up here; unless, of course, we bring them.

Our buddy Pete summed it up perfectly when he joined us for an ascent on Hailey a few weeks ago. "You two have your own Private Idaho out here, don't ya?" It was quite the compliment, comparing Hailey not to the B-52's song but rather to the Idaho side of Teton Pass, some of the best backcountry skiing in the lower forty-eight. No one other than us and a group of our friends have ever skied Mount Hailey. We live in a remote part of Colorado that has more cattle than people. Most of the skiers have settled on the other side of the pass where ski lifts take them to the top of the mountains. People rarely come to our side in the winter and no one would ever think to come back here to ski. No one except my adventurer. He's been skiing Hailey for over twelve years and like the river, knows her every curve. I'm not sure what I've done karmically to deserve this: my own private mountain accompanied by a handsome, sexy guide.

"You go first." He gallantly motions for me to have first tracks.

"I think we should both deflower this virginal meadow simultaneously. A ménage à trois."

He grins as he adjusts the straps on his ski poles. "Three, two, one…" he pauses and delivers the next two words uncharacteristically slow. "Blast. Off."

We launch, skiing side by side, tracing her wide open belly with our turns. She smothers our bodies with soft kisses. We are both driving low into our turns, sliding deep into her, savoring the flow of her across our genitalia. When we weave through her silvery aspen, the blue shadows of her branches drift over our bodies. My spine tingles, my quads burn, the pain and pleasure so exquisitely intertwined. My adventurer is ahead of me, nearing the bottom of the run and I am close, so close. The pain in my legs begs me to stop. I push on, wanting her fully. I initiate my final turn on quivering quads, and get one last thrust before my legs give out and I crash, face first next to our up-track. When I lift my face, it is covered in her juices. I run my tongue all around my lips as my man laughs and reaches out to me.

"Right arm!"

I raise my right hand. He high fives it and helps me up. There is no need to confer about a second lap as we start digging into our packs for our climbing skins. We mount her again and again until we are completely spent. On our final descent, our lust shifts and we start fantasizing about cold beer, tortilla chips and elk burgers back at the cabin.

As my man straps our gear back on the snowmobile, I turn and bow again, this time in gratitude that I am still alive, more so now than ever.

"Thanks, Beauty."

We straddle Black Betty and speed toward the cabin. About a mile out, we stop at a clearing and turn to look back at Mount Hailey. In the muted light of a January afternoon, she glows much like a lover after a wildly satisfying romp. Instead of the slightly swollen lips and tangled hair, she displays the telltale signs of a winter mistress: the curving serpentine tracks of her two most ardent lovers.

CHAPTER FOUR

Early April 2006
Synthesex

RAIN GENTLY DRUMS on the metal roof of our cabin. The April sky is heavy and gray and feels like it has seeped through the window and settled on my eyelids. Mount Hailey is shedding her winter coat and the rivers aren't running yet so I have no mistresses to contend with today. Mud season is in full swing and we have nowhere to go but much to do. We are tucked into our nest hatching dreams.

My lover's arm encircles my waist and pulls me across the sheet until my back is nestled up tight against the warmth of his chest. He nudges my top leg forward with his, enmeshing our genitalia as his face burrows into the hair at the nape of my neck. His bicep cradles my head under our shared pillow and I reach up, interlacing my fingers in his. I marvel at how well we fit, like the last two interlocking pieces of a jigsaw, love no longer a puzzle.

His other hand slides over my hip and gently caresses my thigh before it settles there and becomes still. I lie awake, looking for the faces that live in the wood grain of our aspen ceiling, not wanting to sleep through this dream.

For years, when my previous boyfriend would bolt out of bed at six a.m., I would lie alone and fantasize about this kind of all-encompassing embrace. My man's body is longer and broader than mine, easily surrounding my 5′ 2″ frame. I feel cocooned, snug and warm. We've often joked about how much fun it would be to swap sensations during love making, to experience each other's ecstasy. I wonder if this is how it feels to be inside of me, this sensation of being completely engulfed in love. My hand drifts down next to his and rests on my mound. The pressure of it is comforting and heavy like the clouds.

Outside our bedroom loft window, spring is striving. The aspen branches, teeming with green buds, press up against our window and last week's snowdrifts have morphed into marshy ponds that crackle with the percussive hymns of chorus frogs. Scattered amidst the sage, huddled low and close to the earth, courageous little wildflowers make their debut in blooms of yellow and purple. Inside we are budding as well, our minds steeped and fertile like the muddy earth.

I let my left hand move until I feel his wedding band beneath mine. Our love affair has been an adventurous one, played out amidst mountains and rivers, and driven initially by body and heart. The sex was so mind-blowing there wasn't much of our brains left for any kind of critical thinking. We traded our savings account balances for traveler's checks and flew to New Zealand where we spent two months backpacking through the mountains and plunging our two-person raft through turquoise white water. My lover pounced on me in the middle of a trail run across the Kaikoura peninsula and there, on the earth, framed by ocean and snowy peaks, he proposed. When we landed back in Colorado, we gathered our family and friends, hired a blues band, harvested an elk, and plunged into marriage.

After so many months of neglect, our intellects demanded to be in on the action.

My husband is currently in the throes of a graduate degree in wildlife biology. I am writing like a fiend. We stayed up late last night, glued to our solar-charged laptops. He designed GIS maps to track elk in the San Luis Valley while I encouraged a frustrated couple with fertility issues to mate like a couple of mountain lions. Our thoughts were like a bunch of kids at a slumber party, much too stimulated to sleep. We tossed and turned well past midnight trying to calm them.

I refrain from moving too much now, not wanting to wake up the scientist and the writer just yet. Only my fingers move between my thighs, caressing my petals that are ample and thick like an iris. They become slippery, oozing nectar, blossoming from my touch. I feel him harden and move his erection between my thighs and up against my bud, rubbing our blood-engorged tissues against each other. His lips are moist on my neck as his palm floats across my nipple. I guide him to my entrance and engulf him in my slick, tight embrace.

We are one creature now connected at our cores, our limbs so entangled that I can no longer tell what is his body and what is mine. We slither slowly under the covers, a sleepy, serpentine mass of lust.

I am suddenly hot from this fire we are kindling and just when I'm about to push away some blankets, my lover reaches up and cracks the window, allowing the cool moist morning to drift over us. This has been happening a lot lately. Just as I have a thought, he acts on it. The other day when we were riding in his truck, I felt thirsty and watched as his hand reached down for the water bottle between the seats.

There is a synthesis going on here, activated, I believe, by our lovemaking when we meld into one being like this, encouraging the essence of our fluids to seep into each other's cells. The plants use chlorophyll, sunlight and water. We cultivate with passion. I feel the tendrils of him growing in me when out of the blue I find myself pulling up to a whitewater store to buy a visor for my river helmet. I see the sprouts of me in him when he declared last Saturday a Writing Day. After weeks of training in the mid-day sun, I can run five miles now. As the day fades to dusk, he can sit and meditate for thirty minutes.

Our movements under the covers are unhurried and all about our hips. My lover's hand encourages mine as I rub the heel of it against my clitoris and spread my fingers into a peace sign that slides back and forth around the base of his shaft. We are deep, our spines undulating as one, as our hips rock and sway, enticing our orgasm to rise up and dance with us. When it does, it is slow and dreamy like a waltz.

We roll onto our stomachs and watch the clouds settling on the east ridge of Mount Hailey and listen to the birds who have returned en masse, making our sage meadow sound like a jungle. We are quiet and haven't yet spoken a word. I imagine by the time we are eighty, we won't even need to speak.

I slip down the stairs to make coffee, leaving him to watch the pair of mountain bluebirds that have moved into the box he built for them outside our loft window. When I return, I see it in his eyes: statistics, GIS maps, elk survivability rates. This week he has two final exams and the preliminary draft of his research project is due. I hand him his coffee mug and lie down beside him, already drafting this story in my head.

The rain is hammering down on the roof now, coming down in sheets. Making everything grow.

CHAPTER FIVE

Late April 2006
Fuck Me Fuchsia

I WAKE UP SO PARCHED my lips will surely crack if I dare to smile, which isn't likely. The first thing I see when I look out our bedroom loft window is my man's red truck parked next to the wind generator. I barely notice the peaceful flutter of prayer flags attached to the generator's support cables as my gaze hones in on the dreaded sight of three kayaks strapped to the roof of the truck.

The river has sent her summons. It is time to make good on that promise to share.

I slip downstairs to make coffee and even though I have four lip balms floating around in my life right now, I can't find any of them. What I do find, is my most needy self sitting at the kitchen table looking miserable. She is dressed, as always, in her floor-length, sage-green lace wedding dress. I call her The Pathetic Wife.

"Six weeks." Her voice is something between a sigh and a whimper as she slumps down across the oak table, one arm splaying across it while the other falls over her heart.

"Hey, Drama Queen," I say, trying to keep her from backing into the dark hole of our abandonment issues. "We'll be fine. It's good material. We'll write about it."

I catch her reflection in one of the saucepans hanging above the stove and see tears welling up in her eyes.

"Don't do this. This is our last morning to have sex *for a month and a half,*" I say as I pour two mugs of coffee. "Don't you dare get all miserable and screw everything up. Save the theatrics for after he is gone. *Please...*"

As The Pathetic Wife rests her head on her folded arms with a defeated sigh, I notice a pint of strawberries on the table. I balance them on top of the coffee mugs and head back up to the loft.

My kayaker stirs when he hears the sound of his pottery mug landing on the window sill above his head. I run my hand along the curve of his spine, down into the valley of his low back before letting it settle on the hard mound of his buttocks. He moans and slithers under my touch. I'm about to sink my teeth into one of those firm butt cheeks, when my throat unexpectedly tightens and my eyes tear up.

I look over my shoulder and catch The Pathetic Wife creeping up the stairs.

Get back, I convey through narrowed eyes. If looks could kill she would be dead in a heap on the stairs.

I hide my face in my coffee mug, letting the steam soothe my eyes as I lie on my belly next to my man. We sip in silence as we watch chickadees hop from the bird feeder to the surrounding aspen branches. The leaves are just starting to unfurl, teasing my man whose migration to the California Salmon River every year to run Class V whitewater and teach kayaking makes him miss the vibrant explosion of spring around our love nest. His passion for the river runs deep, so deep, that he leaves me every spring to be with her. I'm learning to share him with the river and in the process have started to fall under her spell as well. But I have to wait six long weeks before I can join him there.

I blink rapidly to flush away the moisture that is pooling around my lower lashes and threatening to trickle down my cheeks. I reach for a strawberry, desperate for distraction. They are red, ripe and luscious, unlike the dead colorless berries I've been paying too much for all winter. As I take a bite, it bursts with juice that is cool and soothing. I rub the soft flesh of the berry back and forth across my lips like a balm until they are dripping and sticky. I roll to my side, facing my husband.

"What do you think? Is it my color?" I ask as I lean over and kiss him.

"Oh, definitely. Freckle face strawberry." He refers to my Irish skin that still gets pink and mottled with freckles, no matter how much sunscreen I use.

"I was thinking of something more seductive..." I lick and suck at my berry before popping the rest of it in my mouth.

He takes the last sip of his coffee and turns on his side, matching my posture by propping his head on the hand of his bent arm.

"Well, I suppose an erotica writer like yourself would only wear the shade Cocksucker Red," he says as his hand reaches down and strokes his erection that is twitching to life.

"Cocksucker Red... I don't know... it's a bit overused. Quickly becoming a cliché, I'm afraid." I take a bite from the middle of an enormous red berry, letting my teeth form a V shape that will snug up perfectly to his expanding cock.

"How about Fruity Fellatio?" I ask as my hand drops down and slides the berry up and down his shaft until it is glistening with a pink, sticky glaze.

He grabs a berry and rubs it against his lips. "I think I'll call mine Cunnilingus Crimson," he says as he proceeds to paint my vulva and labia with it.

We knock heads as we dive simultaneously for the other's juices and laugh and wrestle over who gets to go first. Of course he is bigger and stronger and I am about to get pinned. I'm not interested in waiting for that sticky strawberry cock.

"I've got it, I've got it," I say excitedly.

He lets me win as I push him on to his back. "So here are the rules: when the berry is gone," I say as I bite another one in half and let the red juice dribble on his chest, "it's the other person's turn. No orgasms. If you feel one coming on you say, 'Ding'."

"Ding?" he says with a laugh as he watches me draw the curve of a ski track down his belly.

"Yeah, 'ding', like a timer going off. And then the other person gets to go. I'll go first and show you how it works."

He lies back. "If I must....

I lick the juices from his chest and belly and slowly descend to his cock that is hard, sticky and pink like a Popsicle. I lean down and lick it once from the base to the tip. The heat of his arousal has warmed the strawberry juice enhancing its sweetness. He tastes so good that I find myself slurping and sucking him from every angle until he is clean. I grab my berry and douse him with more juice and begin to suck hard with my lips before sliding him down my throat as my hand jacks up and down the base of his shaft.

"Ding," he says with a moan.

I lift my sticky face to him as he grabs a berry, rubs it on my lips and kisses me.

"Hmm, now that's a great shade. I think I'll call it Deep Throat Maroon," he says as he guides me on my back and saturates the fleshy folds of my sex until I am dripping and ripe. He sucks and licks, devouring my fruit like he is starving. I feel myself starting to quiver.

"Ding." I pull his face up to mine. "Mmmmm…Strawberry Pussy Puree," I say as I taste the sweet musky mix of flavors on his lips.

"Testicle Tickling Shimmer," I announce as I push him down on his back and rub a berry all over his scrotum. I tickle his testicles with my sticky fingers while I lick and suck them clean. It doesn't take long.

"Ding."

We are playing like a couple of kids on a seesaw, up and down, his head between my legs, mine between his, giggling and laughing as we suck each other to the brink. At times like this, I feel like we are eight years old. But with all the perks of adulthood: cars, credit cards and our very own tree fort.

He grabs a berry and rubs it on my nipples.

"Berry Breast Ecstasy," he says proudly as he teases and licks them with his tongue. "Eat Me Mauve," he announces as he dives back down.

I am squirming, laughing. And so close. "Ding!"

"Ass Tickling Temptation," I say as I slowly twirl a berry until the green stem pops off. He smiles and lies back as I pull his sticky cock deep into my throat and let my berry dance around his anus which is sure to put him over the edge.

"Ding," he says, his voice strained from trying so hard to control his orgasm.

He pushes me back on the bed and grabs a berry.

"Bad Girl Burgundy." He circles the berry around on my clit. I know I will explode if his tongue follows. I reach up and grab the last berry and rub it wildly all over my lips before throwing my arms open wide.

"Fuck Me Fuchsia!" I am having so much fun, laughing so hard that I don't notice The Pathetic Wife slipping into our bed.

My husband's sculpted forearms are on either side of my head as he slowly lowers his body into mine. His brown eyes are hooded and intense, reminding me of one of the Salmon River osprey honing in on its prey. I feel the thickness of him penetrating me, filling me, completing me. And then it hits me.

This is the last time for a long time.

"Six weeks..." I say as my eyes fill. His do too.

We are no longer eight-year-olds. We are forty-something, passionate and filled with the longing we will be managing for the next month and a half. The poignancy of our impending farewell intensifies the sensation of every stroke, every kiss, every thrust. We are desperate to fill ourselves with each other, as if we can store and ration this passion.

I lift my torso and wrap my legs around his waist as he pulls me close until our hearts feel like they are beating in one chest. His hands drop, cupping my buttocks as he pulses my body into his. I squeeze and tighten around him, conveying with my body what I won't let myself say.

Don't go, don't go, don't go.

I wrap my arms tightly around his neck and pull him even deeper into me, wanting him so far inside me that he'll never find his way out.

With each pulse, he penetrates the place where I stuff the things I don't want to feel. With each thrust, everything I've been trying to suppress—the sadness, the longing, the fear that I may never see him again—begins to break loose. Emotional repression isn't selective. By trying to put a lid on my sadness, I've also cut myself off from my bliss. As he urges his body into mine, he sets them both free. They intertwine with the sensation of a hundred little strawberry seeds rubbing against my clit before rising up and exploding like a geyser at my throat, a release so intense that there is no room for breath, leaving me gasping and sobbing. The ecstasy of loving him blends so exquisitely with the grief of having to let him go that I can no longer tell them apart. When he climaxes, I am propelled even higher. This prompts another wave of tears coupled with hysterical laughter. I bite down on my lip and taste blood, metallic and bitter. As I lick it away, I taste the berries, juicy and sweet.

I wipe away my tears with trembling, sticky fingers as my husband caresses my back in long, soothing strokes.

'Wow," I say when I can finally talk.

"Those Farewell Fucks…"

"You ought to go away more often," I say through choked laughter.

"Well, you know, the only thing better than a Farewell Fuck…"

I look at him perplexed. What could possibly be better than this?

"…is the reuniting one."

He speaks softly as if he is telling me a fairy tale.

"Six weeks from now we'll be curling up together on the beach at the Salmon River…"

As he talks my head is filled with images. The warm, heavy air filled with the sound of crickets. My naked body cradled in the sand beneath our sleeping bags. The silhouette of his head, ink-black against the sparkling backdrop of the Milky Way, hovering featureless above me.

The sound of the river, cooing in my ear, as they both flow into me.

CHAPTER SIX

May 2006
Holding My Own

I AM SITTING NAKED on the deck of my cabin watching a May morning unfold on my winter-white skin. My kayaker is in California making love to his favorite river for six weeks. In his absence, I've taken a few lovers of my own.

I bring the soles of my feet together and lean forward, letting the weight of my elbows push my knees into my yoga mat. The radiant hand of Sun slides down the cobbled path of my vertebrae before he penetrates my low back and cleft with his heat. As I exhale, my pelvic floor melts, flooding my canal with warmth.

Wind, barely a breeze this early, lightly tickles my moist, splayed labial lips. I sink deeper into my forward bend, wishing I was flexible enough to kiss him there. I settle for resting my forehead on my ankles and inhaling the co-mingled fragrance of my sex and the sodden earth that is swirling around the diamond-shaped bowl of my bent legs. I hold the stretch, intoxicated by the brew, until a light burning in the muscles of my lower back urges me to flow onward.

I straighten my spine and lift my torso until I can feel Wind awakening further to stroke my breasts. I run my pinky finger across my tongue, moisten it, and draw a spiraling path around my areola for him to follow. When he does, his touch, still cool and reminiscent of night, makes me shiver as my nipples harden. I spread my legs wide, arch my spine backwards and open myself to Sun, letting him drench me with his yellow tongue. I feel a flush of heat as he licks me from my vulva to my chin. Wind follows Sun's swath with cool insistent kisses that dimple my skin, sending an orgasmic chill across my flesh.

My hand drifts down across the plateau of my belly and floats like a pendulum, back and forth across my mound, enticing my lovers there. I separate my folds, exposing myself to them. The combination of Wind's chill and Sun's ardor is icy hot on my erect bud, like menthol. I shudder as the sensation permeates my sex and vibrates up my spine.

I pause and breathe, savoring the small spasms of pleasure that are as delicate and sweet as the wildflowers blooming all around me. I lie on my back, encouraging more tremors with my fingers and inhale deeply, engaging my breath as a vehicle to transport this ecstasy through my entire body. My skin tingles from my scalp to my toes.

I thrust my feet up toward the sky before lowering them behind my head for plow pose, stretching my hamstrings, my hips, my sex. I spread my legs and gush as my lovers simultaneously caress my offering. My fingers reach, interlace with theirs, and begin drumming against my wet, swollen lips, sending percussive vibrations echoing down my sheath. I hold the pose, savoring the quivering at my cervix before sliding two fingers in to greet it.

My sheath responds immediately, clenching rhythmically around my fingers. I hold the pose for just a moment before I succumb to the urge to pulse. Sun and Wind dance at my entrance, warming me and cooling me, each time my fingers emerge from my slippery canal.

My neck begins to feel less than ecstatic, so I lower my legs and flow forward into a seated forward bend. As I try to catch the breath that I lost somewhere in my last orgasm, I sway my body from side to side, letting my nipples graze across my thighs as Wind plays with the hair that has unwound from the single braid that hangs thick and heavy down my back. As Sun rises higher in the sky, his intensity, coupled with my arousal and the rising vigor of my practice, makes me sweat. The backs of my thighs are damp and sticky against the squishy foam of my yoga mat, my sex, like a marsh wedged between.

I roll over on to my belly and place my hands on either side of my breasts, letting my thumbs gently brush the edges of my nipples. I drive my clit downward, grounding my pelvis, and then slowly unpeel the tacky flesh of my belly from the mat as I lift my torso into cobra pose. My head rolls from side to side and I giggle as Wind tickles my face with the wisps of blond hair that have escaped the tether of my braid. I roll my shoulders back and push my chest forward and up to Sun, opening my heart to him as I begin to pulse my clit against the hardness of the wood deck beneath my mat. I hold the pose, and inhale the unbridled essence of my lovers deep into my lungs, letting the vitality of spring permeate my every cell.

My clit begins to quiver as do the muscles of my arms that are starting to feel the strain of maintaining this posture. I continue to hold, savoring the sensation of every muscle spasm—the ones of pleasure, the ones of exertion—until heat rises from my core and explodes across my chest. A trickle of sweat drips down my ribcage, its path quickly cooled by Wind. Hot tears flow down my cheeks and before I have a chance to contemplate their origins, Wind wipes them away, telling me there is no need for definition. Everything is flowing: blood, breath, sweat, tears, and I allow it all, for as long as I can, before lowering my torso down on to the mat.

I roll onto my back, completing my practice with stillness. As I slow my breath, I feel Wind and Sun settle in beside me. I relax in Savasana, also known as the corpse pose. Funny that name, because I feel so incredibly alive.

I hold the pose.

CHAPTER SEVEN

May-June 2006
Buck Me

DAY ONE: MAY IS BARELY blooming in the Colorado high country which means the rivers are roaring to life in Northern California. My kayaker is driving west, moving farther from me with each beat of my heart. To distract myself, I clean the cabin, reclaiming the space that will be mine alone for the next six weeks. He has left little bits of himself scattered around the cabin like crumbs: a pile of screws, a wool sock, outdated wildlife journals, ski wax. As I tuck his things away, I notice something hairy behind the couch and discover a rumpled antelope hide. I shake it out and spread it on the deck, letting the spring sun revive its wild, leathery scent.

Day Seven: I've been meditating twice a day on the deck watching our ski tracks dissolve into Mt. Hailey as she trades her winter coat for an aspen leaf skirt. Whenever my thoughts wander, I am lured back to the meadow in front of me that is eight different shades of green and blooming with glacier lilies and bluebells. As if the mountain is my personal meditation coach, she whispers in my ear: *Stay here, right here. Why would you want to be anywhere else when you are surrounded by so much beauty?*

Day Eight: Can you fall in love with a piece of land? I feel such an intimacy with our 120-acre property when I am alone here. As if the surrounding peaks know my man is gone, they keep me busy like concerned girlfriends. Mount Hailey hangs out with me while I meditate and do yoga on the deck. Ute Peak entices me to trail run on her soft muddy trails brimming with sagebrush and mule deer. The vista where we got married invites me over for sunset hikes and provides a portal for me to launch love and intentions westward to my kayaker.

Day Nine: I am enjoying not sharing my body. I don't shave my legs. My hair is in a perpetual greasy ponytail. I've been lounging around the cabin for two days rotating between running clothes and the same pair of yoga pants and T-shirt. Since I don't need to be clean for my lover, I am steeping in my own humus-like scent. My laptop doesn't seem to mind.

Day Ten: The energy of spring is about waking up and as the earth emerges from her long winter nap, I, too, feel like I am rubbing sleep from my eyes. Even though I miss my man, I achieve a level of bliss that isn't possible when he is here. Since he isn't around to frost with all my love and adoration, I find myself sitting with a big bowl of icing and I'm the only cake in sight. I am reading a book by Sylvia Boorstein, *That's Funny, You Don't Look Buddhist*. She confesses that through her exploration of meditation she unexpectedly fell in love with herself. Her words resonate like the thunder of this afternoon's rainstorm.

Day Fifteen: I've had some visitors. As the snow continues to melt, the animals have reclaimed the high country and seem to have a migratory path through our property. A cow moose and her twin calves have been hanging out in the willows by the creek. I do my best to avoid the herd of elk that uses Ute Peak as a nursery, although they don't seem to mind my presence. I feel quieter, calmer, and wonder if my energy is now vibrating at a frequency more in sync with theirs. The hummingbirds love my magenta bikini and buzz my breasts when I am lying with my heart stretched to the sky in fish pose. Yesterday, a butterfly landed on my shoulder while I sipped a cup of green tea. I felt like Snow White.

Day Sixteen: I thought I was doing just fine with celibacy, approaching it as a spiritual practice and channeling my longing into writing. And I do have a blast tapping into this part of myself who is one of my favorite persons to hang out with. The only problem is she doesn't have a cock.

Sure, I love this solitude, this place of love that emanates from within and isn't dependent on someone else. I wouldn't feel this if he was here and I wouldn't explore the longing that drives these erotic stories.

But still, if I let my thoughts drift—and I can't seem to stop them today—I miss him desperately, deeply, in my core. I crave the hard maleness of him. I crave the softness of his moist lips and the way his smile tilts to the left and lifts one eyebrow after he climaxes. The earth needs to scream today to bring me back to my breath and away from my fantasies of him. I keep reminding myself that this longing is a gift and I am lucky to feel so much love for another person.

I realize I'm rambling here but this is a diary so there's implied permission. I'm not sure exactly what my point is, but I do know this: today I would willingly trade my whole bowl of icing for one taste of him.

Day Nineteen: I am running through mud, which is a perfect analogy for how my writing felt this morning. But as I climb the winding trails of Ute Peak, my legs are like a pump, drawing up the words and images that were mired in muck at my keyboard. I stop and pull a damp piece of paper and a small pencil from my sports bra trying to collect the words:

...he moans, making my sheath salivate like one of Pavlov's dogs...wanting him so deep inside of me he'll never find his way out.

I've already run three miles and since I'm primed now to write, I turn back instead of finishing the eight-mile loop. When I do, I run into a coyote standing in my muddy footprints. He is beautiful, like a small wolf. I have never understood why people regard these wild canines with such disdain. He doesn't seem the least bit surprised when we meet on the trail. I have a sense that he's been tracking the pungent tang of my sweat that smells like the wild game that I eat. Or perhaps he's been lured by the scent of pheromones undoubtedly oozing out my pores. I reach slowly into my sports bra, pull out my pencil and paper and start scribbling down some notes. When I look up he is gone.

Day Twenty: I wake up at dawn to the sound of a gong. I wonder if my brain is getting so conditioned to meditating in the morning that it thinks we are at an ashram.

I lie still thinking maybe it's time to drop the purifying rituals and have a cup of coffee and a cigarette when I hear the sound again outside my window. When I look out I see the culprit: a male blue grouse pumping his throat and spreading his plumage. He is courting a brown-feathered female who blends so exquisitely into the earth I can barely see her. She scurries away from him toward the back of the cabin. I run downstairs and move from window to window watching. I know I'm projecting, but I can't help but wonder: why the hell is she running away?

Day Twenty-One: I am naked and holding cobra pose on the deck, savoring the warmth of the morning sun on my skin. Something hot releases in my chest and tears trickle down my cheeks and between my breasts. I still have fourteen days until I go to California to see him and suddenly two weeks feels like an eternity. I hold the pose until I am shaking.

Still Day Twenty-One: I keep reminding myself that I choose this solitude. I could invite friends out to the cabin to join me, but I don't. Women, we can't help ourselves, we talk, and talk. I can't invite any of my male friends out here with all this sex-deprived, erotic energy bouncing off the log walls.

Writing and meditation are, after all, solitary sports. My meditation practice hasn't felt very sporty lately though, more like a wolf in sheep's clothing. After three weeks, the soft fluffy coat is molting, exposing fangs. The image of myself as a cool independent woman who can let her husband go chase whitewater is nowhere in sight. When I see my reflection in the sliding glass door, I see a needy, angry shrew.

Day Twenty-Three: I don't know why they call it the path of enlightenment. I feel so heavy today. I don't meditate. I don't write. Instead, I read a bestseller, eat tortilla chips between naps on the couch and watch two movies on my laptop.

Day Twenty-Six: I remember reading that there are two base emotions that all others rise from: love and fear. Well, this isn't love that I am feeling. My husband has a week off from teaching at the kayak school and is paddling a Class V river for the next three days. I worry about him, which I know is a static that I don't want to extend out to the universe. I hike up to our wedding vista, add a rock to the cairn where we exchanged our vows and send out a better intention:

May he be safe. May he be safe. May he be safe.

Day Twenty-Seven: The Pathetic Wife is out of control. She has saved all his phone messages—twelve so far—and listens to them one after another. This ritual is twisted, I know, but if the river ever decides to swallow him whole at least I will still have his voice. I use the same justifying logic when I write out those health insurance checks: if I have it, I won't need it.

But there was one message in particular where his voice dropped an octave at the end when he said: *I miss you.* The longing came crashing through my keeping-busy barrier like a flash flood, pinning me against the wall. Wanting to drown in it, I slid down until I was level with the answering machine at my yoga studio and hit the repeat button so hard I cracked my fingernail. Every cell in my body leaned toward the speaker to better hear the intonation of desire in his voice, to better hear those three simple words that unstitch me and my illusion that it is okay that I haven't seen or touched him in a month.

Day Twenty-Eight: I haven't had any alcohol since he left and I've proved, like Sandra Bullock when she portrayed an alcoholic going through rehab, that I too can go twenty-eight days without it. Celibacy and sobriety at the same time are proving to be excessive, so I decide to have a glass of white wine on the deck as the sun begins to set. I've dug into the musical archives and am listening to the band *Everything But the Girl*, swinging my foot to their '80s techno groove when the song *Missing* comes on:

And I miss you

Like the deserts miss the rains

My swinging foot lands on the deck as the music pulls me from my chair. I played this song two years ago, the first time I stripped for my husband. I wrote him a play, a role play actually, and unwrapped myself for his Christmas present. I stayed within our $50 spending limit by scoring impossibly high-heeled shoes at a thrift store and a lacy red bra and matching thong at Target. In the script, he was the recently divorced grad student who gets dragged to a strip club by his office mate and promptly falls for me, the melancholy erotic dancer who wraps her legs and her longing around her dance pole. I improvised by using the aspen support log under the loft.

I haven't heard this song since that night and suddenly I am recreating my role, dancing slowly, seductively with my longing. I feel like a desert, my desire so vast, stretching out like the Sahara for another week. I'm thirsty for him, his moist kisses on my neck, his wet tongue between my thighs.

The setting sun dances with me, reaching her fiery arms across the sky. I raise my hands over head and grasp her magnificent, orange fingers and spin beneath her, undulating my hips to the rhythms of the song's drum machine. A breeze tickles my ankle and rises up my legs and stomach. I pull off my T-shirt. My bra follows.

Could you be dead

Always were two steps ahead

I feel tears pooling in my eyes, so I push away the lyrics, push away the fear. I fill in my own words.

May he be safe in the sun

All the hard whitewater done

I imagine him relaxing on the beach after a hard day of paddling, feeling my longing and love radiating down on him through the rays of his California sunset. He closes his eyes and gets a vision of me sliding my hands across my breasts and down my abdomen as they push away my cutoffs and thong. I release my ponytail so my hair falls freely down my back. I can feel his lustful gaze scanning up and down my body as the breeze blows wisps of hair across my face.

I am naked, eyes closed, arms poised overhead. My head falls back and my eyes open, taking in the magnificence of the day's final rays stretching across the sky, enticing the three quarter moon as it rises from behind Ute Peak.

I lower my gaze and I am stunned into stillness by a buck antelope standing across the meadow watching me. He is beautiful. The black of his horns looks as if it has bled down to his snout, shrouding his face in a dark mask. His hide, in contrast, is light, streaks of tan and white stretched tight across his striated ribs and muscular haunches. He exudes pure unadulterated maleness.

I hold my writhing goddess pose not wanting to startle him, not wanting him to leave. The song, the last of the play list, ends. The only sound is my ragged breath.

He lifts his snout to the breeze and smells me: the sweet tang of wine on my breath, the ripe muskiness of my sex. He takes one step closer and then another. I can almost differentiate a pair of eyes, black as a new moon night, appraising me.

I am still as a leafless tree, my arms extended overhead like branches, but they are burning from the effort and I have to lower them. My movement breaks the spell. He bolts across the meadow and becomes a blur as my eyes swell with tears. I blink fast to clear them, but he is already gone.

Inside, I take the antelope hide up to the loft and drape it over the banister next to my bed.

Still Day Twenty-Eight: It is almost midnight and I can't sleep. One glass of wine and my head is buzzing. The May moon radiates in my loft window casting the cabin in an ethereal, insomniac glow. My uterus is waxing like the moon and I feel like a lunatic, wired and hormonal.

If my husband were here, I would amuse myself by stroking his back while he slept, tracing the strong mound of his buttocks and toying with his soft, sleepy cock until it hardened in my hand. But he isn't here and he hasn't been for a month and tonight I can no longer make any sense of it. Five weeks is too long. I feel abandoned and pissed off.

I can't go find sex or companionship anywhere else because I am married. But I don't feel married because my husband is nowhere in sight. So I am fucked. Or rather not fucked.

My palm drifts down to my wild bush that hasn't been trimmed in a month. I tap, releasing the ripe scent of my sex like pollen. My fingers explore, spreading my petals, exposing my bud. Suddenly, I am so sick of all this soft feminine energy, all this taking care of myself. I want a shot of whiskey, a three-day beard scraping against my cheek, a hard cock. I slap my sex once, twice, but it does nothing for me.

I fall into a restless sleep thinking about the buck, his dark, mysterious face and how amazing it felt to be seen.

Barely Day Twenty-Nine: I am running through an early morning snowstorm when the buck suddenly appears amidst the sage. He is standing in profile, forming a dark silhouette against the muted light of the rising sun. He has been waiting, the fastest male on earth, as still as a bronzed statue, just for me. He turns to face me and the intensity of his black gaze drops me to my knees.

I want him to get closer. I want to smell his musky animal scent. I want to get lost in the dark of those eyes.

He rakes a front hoof across the snow. His breath billows from his snout like steam. We are about twenty feet apart. I hold still despite my nearly overwhelming urge to move towards him. A wiser part of me warns and holds back.

Let him come to you.

He does, charging forward with dark horns that could easily eviscerate me.

Don't move.

I don't. He halts within two feet, appraising me with that dark mask as if I passed some kind of test for not moving. He hooves the ground near me, snorts and moves closer. I know he can smell me, my salty sweat, my gushing sex. He smells wild, of wet earth, sage and musk. His hide is dank from the snow, coarse, and the color of caramel and vanilla ice cream. My hand trembles at my side itching to touch him.

Don't.

My yearning overrides my intuition this time and I extend my hand. He lowers his head encouragingly, I think, but then suddenly he rears up, his front hooves clamoring together above my head as if he is scrambling for purchase on the snowy air. I fall back trembling, and watch in amazement as he lands, transformed, his head and torso now morphed into a man.

My man.

The dark hair on my husband's chest flows like a stream down his sculpted abdomen right into the tawny muscled shoulders of the buck. My man's familiar brown eyes have replaced the antelope's black ones, but the horns remain, an extension of his dark hair. I stand still, stunned by the magnificence of my centaur lover. Before I have a chance to fully process it all, a pack of coyotes begin howling like Ute warriors preparing for war. Their cries echo all around us and suddenly, even though my eyes are open, everything is black.

I am alone, belly down in my bed, my hands gripping my pillow so hard my fingers ache.

No, no ,no.

I squeeze my eyes shut.

Come back, come back, come back.

Out of my blurred peripheral vision I see my man's torso suspended horizontally in the air as if he is doing triangle pose in front of the log railing that surrounds our loft. I push up on hands and knees and reach out, desperate to touch his dark pelt and instead feel the coarse wiry hair of the antelope hide. My brain is confused, teetering, and when it finally lands, I am awake with the understanding that my husband is still gone. The weight of the realization is so heavy that my arms can no longer hold me. The coyotes are still going off outside my window, laughing hysterically at me, and my dream of a centaur lover. I pull the window closed, mute their heckling and curse them for waking me.

I kick away my blankets, pull the antelope hide over the bare skin of my back and try to summon up the image of my centaur as I push my hands beneath me, cupping my sex. The wooden chest beside the bed houses a vibrator, but I know that every conscious thought, every wakeful movement takes me farther away from my dream.

Come back, come back, come back.

I turn my head and grab the edge of the hide in my teeth, feel the hair stiff against my lips. The hide is warm and heavy against my haunches and feels as if my centaur is back preparing to mount me. I push my face against the wood banister imagining one of his horns, dangerously close to my cheek. Even though he is half antelope, I decide my centaur is hung like a horse. While one hand massages my clit, I stack the fingers of the other to form a thick triangular probe.

My dream lover is a compilation of the fastest animal on earth merged with my man who hasn't been inside me for almost five weeks. Coitus isn't going to be a slow, luxurious thing and I don't want it to be. I penetrate myself and thrust wildly, like an antelope surrounded by a band of coyotes would do. His hooves scrape my shoulders where the edge of the hide rubs. I reach up with one hand and grab the banister, caressing his horns, and he thrusts even deeper. I buck back, pushing my hips into the hide as I ride fingers coated with coarse strands of antelope hair that poke and tickle my clit. My cunt begins to shudder as I grunt and buck. As the hide slips off my back, I feel the departing caress of his snout down my spine that dimples my flesh and sends an orgasmic chill out to every neuron in my body. I pull the hide to my chest, hugging and caressing it. It smells wet, like the antelope in my dream dusted with snow. I realize it is wet from tears just before I fall into a deep, dreamless sleep

Day Thirty: When I awaken, morning is flowing like molten lava over Ute Peak and seeping into my bed. As I lounge in bed remembering my romp with my centaur lover, a realization dawns on me as vividly as the sky. It wasn't just a dream.

My husband and that buck *are* the same animal. Tethering him to me would be synonymous to putting an antelope in a cage. He would more likely die from that kind of love than any Class V rapid.

I rest my chin on the windowsill and let the yellowing light warm my face. Only five more days.

I look down and see a dusting of fresh snow on the ground, marred by a single set of hoof tracks.

CHAPTER EIGHT

June 2006
Class V Fantasy

AFTER THIRTY-FIVE DAYS APART, my lover and I are sleeping together again and unfortunately I mean that quite literally. After fourteen-hour workdays teaching beginners how to paddle whitewater, my kayak instructor is exhausted.

But it is Wednesday afternoon at the Otter Bar Kayak School and Lodge and today, under the guise of giving the students a break in the rigorous schedule (the instructors are the ones who need it), is a rest day. This means that after three days of quickies before his 7:30 a.m. instructor meetings, my man will be off the river by 4:00 and we'll have two whole hours to pleasure each other before he returns to the lodge for dinner with the students.

The mosquito netting is draped like a fairy's canopy over the queen-size bed that sits on the deck of the house where we are staying. The owners of this house, that everyone refers to as Outer Bar because it is tucked in the woods at the outer edge of the lodge property, graciously let the lodge and its employees use it when they aren't here. I've supplied the wood headboard with a few mid-summer fuck fest essentials: a mini bar bottle of Grand Marnier, a bowl of fresh sweet cherries, and massage oil. I'm sipping a glass of Pinot Noir in a halter bikini of the same color, communing with my husband's favorite mistress until he gets here.

I must admit, he has great taste. The California Salmon River is exquisite. For starters, there's her warm, emerald-colored water adorned with turquoise swimming holes, languid waterfalls and frothy white rapids. If that isn't enough to make you wet, the narrow, single-lane road that winds for hours through national forest to get to here is rimmed with pink, puffy-lipped sweet peas that look like they are reaching from the shoulder of the road to kiss you. In some locations, white phallic-shaped flowers that resemble lilacs, dangle from above as if botanical fellatio is imminent in the middle of the road. A commune that sprouted here in the sixties still thrives, drawing free spirits who relax naked along her shores, completely comfortable in their own tanned skin.

As long as I'm not upside down in a kayak struggling to roll back up, I love this place. So this year during my annual conjugal visit, I decided to skip the kayak lessons. I've been doing yoga on the beach with the river every morning, biking along her curving road and plunging naked into her deep swimming holes. My skin is browner, my hair blonder, than when I arrived four days ago. I feel saturated with the sensuality of her.

When I hear the crunch of madrone leaves underfoot, I know before I even look up that I will see the bronzed chest and abs of my lover funneling into the black river shorts he left in this morning. His dark hair will be messy from the river running her fingers through it all day. But when I look up I see two bare chests walking towards me through the woods.

My adventurer and I are no strangers to threesomes. We have them all the time with rivers and mountains. But we haven't *yet* had a threesome with another person.

Of course we fantasize about it. After many playful discussions, we've agreed that a stranger would be best, someone we would never see again. A woman. Our best scenario so far is to wander the streets of the red-light district in Amsterdam and let ourselves be seduced by an exotic Indonesian beauty behind one of those sliding glass doors. Never have we seriously entertained the idea of including a friend. Never has our fantasy included a guy.

So I'm not sure what to think when my lover shows up for our sex date with his buddy and fellow kayak instructor, Dave, grinning beside him.

I bring my wine glass to my lips and look over the rim at the two chiseled torsos approaching.

"I know I'm interrupting a fuck date," Dave says, as only Dave could say, as he steps up on the deck. His New Zealand accent and blue eyes caress me first before his arms can get close enough to pull me into a full-body hug. As our bodies meld, he lets out a low, barely discernable moan. Not only is this man an expert kayaker, he is a Class V flirt. "But I'm heading out tomorrow and I don't know when I'll get another chance to see you," he says as he steps back, his hands resting lightly on my shoulders. "You look fabulous."

Part of his charm is when he delivers that kind of compliment, he does it so sincerely that there is no doubt in your mind that it is true. The man defines charisma so I'm not disappointed to see him, ever, even now when the lower half of my otherwise dry bikini is so sopping wet that I keep my thighs pressed together in case I'm leaking through, which, of course only makes me hotter and wetter. Dave is a blond version of my husband in that he is equally passionate about rivers, outdoor adventure and sex. He's an engaging, clever Kiwi, the kind of guy that compliments you on your yoga pants, asks if you are wearing underwear and next thing you know you are going into great detail about your v-string and loosening your drawstring to show him.

As I said, Class V.

"I've been waiting all day," I say as his hands slide slowly down my arms completing our embrace. "I *think* I can wait another fifteen minutes." I kiss my man as he tops off my glass of wine and tosses Dave a cold beer. As we settle on to the deck overlooking the river, the conversation drifts, as it inevitably does here, to kayaking.

My mind drifts, as it inevitably does here, to sex. A threesome with two men has never been a big fantasy of mine, but it doesn't take long before I'm visualizing the three of us sprawled beneath the mosquito netting, Dave at my head, kissing the lips of my mouth upside down like in the Spiderman movie, my head resting in his palms while his fingertips massage the muscles at the base of my skull. My man is kissing the lips between my thighs, my pelvis cradled in his hands as he kneads my gluts. The image has me crossing my legs to contain the latest gush and sends a visible shiver across my skin.

My man notices the goose bumps spreading across my arms and legs. "Are you chilled?" he asks, even though it is ninety degrees on this eve of the summer solstice. He wraps his arm over my shoulder and pulls me closer to him on the couch. I adjust my posture so I am sitting with one leg bent, the foot pressed against my inner thigh now for containment. I feign a yogic spine-straightening move and push my heel into my aching clit.

I sigh and take a sip of wine, savoring it and the exquisite torture of my fantasy before I realize that the conversation has stopped and they are both looking at me.

"What?" I feel my face flush.

"I just asked if you enjoyed your day," Dave says with a smirk as if he can read every lusty little thought that is playing through my mind.

"It was great...and just keeps getting better," I say as my hand floats over and caresses the hair on the back of my man's head. In my fantasy, I love being the object of their intense kayaker focus but the images of it are so arousing, so distracting, that I can hardly talk. I certainly can't handle being the focus of the conversation. I quickly deflect.

"How's fatherhood?" I ask.

Dave's smile gets so big I wonder if his face can contain it. He and his wife Clare, another kayaker who instructs here, took on the ultimate adventure of parenthood last year. They are here this summer with their now six-month-old daughter.

"Fucking amazing," he says confirming what his smile already told me. He starts telling us about the birth. I heard about it through e-mails last January and it sounded pretty scary. The words 'ruptured placenta' are too painful for my current hedonistic state so my thoughts go scurrying back beneath the mosquito netting, where the three of us are kneeling on the bed now.

My man and I are chest to chest, as his erection slides slowly, gloriously, into my long awaiting wetness. We remain still, savoring the communion. I feel the heat, the hardness of Dave behind me. The natural porn flick progression here would be double penetration but when I try to nudge my fantasy there, it won't budge. I'm not a big fan of anal sex and the intensity of two incredibly strong, passionate kayakers thrusting simultaneously inside of me sounds like it would surely split me in two. I click forward on my fantasy remote control.

In this scene, my man is entering me from behind while I take Dave in my mouth, but I mean, really, how could I give an amazing blowjob (and I'd want it to be amazing) while being rocked from behind? Too distracting. Unless…the cadence of my man's thrusts, slow and sultry at first, would provide the rhythm for my fellatio.

I take a sip of wine while I ponder this. On this side of the deck the conversation is back to kayaking and where in California Dave, Clare and their daughter will travel on their upcoming week off from teaching. On the other side, I am kneeling on the bed facing the headboard, gripping it for support. My man kneels behind me, his hands squeezing the flesh of my hips as he slides in. Our legs are splayed, straddled across Dave who lies beneath us on his back. There is a pillow beneath his head that positions his lips and tongue at the perfect height of my sex. His hands have easy access to my hard nipples. Each thrust drives my clit into Dave's eagerly awaiting tongue and lips. Each thrust flattens my nipples against Dave's arousingly rough, calloused hands. My cervix quivers on both sides of the deck.

I lean into my man wondering, would he go for it? Would he want to share his wife with another guy? Do I want him to want to?

And what about Dave? I remember a conversation last summer when he told me about a life-changing moment he had while kayaking a Class V stretch of river. "All of a sudden it dawned on me that my pregnant wife and unborn child were waiting for me in New Zealand," he said. "For the first time in my life I wondered what the hell I was doing." Since then I think he has toned down the kayaking and the flirting, for that matter, to Class IV.

But even if both of them were willing to go for it, there's this little bitty issue of Dave's wife Clare. She's one of the coolest women on the planet and the reason that Dave's expert flirting never gets out of hand. None of the women around here would ever cross a sexual boundary with Dave because we have so much respect for Clare. Furthermore, if Dave ever hurt her, all his friends would disown him. So, we'd have to get her blessing which I am sure after nursing and changing dirty nappies all day, she'd willingly give. The guys are laughing about some antic of one of the rookie instructors now and I join in as I imagine the three of us running through the woods to the instructors' cabin so Dave could use the phone to call Clare. "Hey, love, I'm going to be late for dinner. Just hanging out for an after work shag."

But even if we made it through that hurdle, I hear the voice of Creek, the head instructor and patriarch of our tribe of Salmon River kayakers. One night around a bonfire we got him talking about the commune days. "We tried open relationships and the whole free love thing in the sixties. There was just too much jealousy and resentment. Believe me, it didn't work."

I hear an empty beer bottle land on the table. Dave stands up, and like a gymnast that has just landed a double backflip, his arms open emphatically.

"Have a fabulous fuck."

I feel like telling him that we just did. All three of us. But instead, the three of us embrace and laugh at his parting remark. Only on the Salmon River.

My kayaker takes my hand and leads me towards the other side of the deck. As he does, I can't help but wonder if Dave is really going home or if he loops back through the woods for some harmless Class III voyeurism.

CHAPTER NINE

July 2006
Drill Me, Baby Drill Me

I WAKE UP WET.

It is dark, sometime between midnight, when we finally put down our weapons, and dawn, when we crawl out of bed and pick them back up. Our hands, empty for this brief interim, take advantage of our sleepy semiconscious state to reach across the sheets for each other.

In the waking hours they are too busy waging war to make love.

Ten days ago we learned that the mineral rights for 41,000 acres of land in our pristine county are going up for auction for oil and gas development. Our cabin and its surrounding acreage are included in the sale. When I saw the article in the local paper, I called my kayaker in California and read it to him over the phone. He called back the next day and said he was coming home.

"You are leaving the Salmon River at the height of kayak season?" I was stunned. I didn't think anything was *that* important.

"This is bad. Really bad." His voice sounded thick. "Our property is part of an old homestead. We don't own the mineral rights. And if its coal bed methane they're after..." He didn't finish the sentence. He didn't have to. The mailing address for our property is Coalville. "I'm leaving in the morning."

I hung up the phone and did a search on coal bed methane. The articles I read made my stomach clench. My husband, my marriage, our secluded off-the-grid cabin have been a dream come true. If an oil and gas company bought our mineral rights and started drilling, it could very quickly turn into a nightmare.

George W. and Cheney are in the White House, an oil administration if there ever was one. Right now the laws favor oil and gas development, a policy that hopefully, for the sake of the environment, will shift with the next election. The oil and gas companies know this and are snatching up leases now. If they buy the lease on our property, they have the legal right to build roads, house employees, and erect drilling rigs every ten acres. As I keep reading, I learn more about the methods of extracting coal bed methane which involves pulling all the groundwater out to release the gas. If that isn't bad enough for the already parched West, there is the issue of the contaminated waste water. After I read about the impact this has on creek, fish and wildlife ecology, I don't sleep much that night.

When my activist gets home the next day, there is no passionate Reuniting Fuck. This isn't about us.

We meet at our colorful, but crooked old house in town where my healing arts and yoga studio live, and set up our command post. We have six days to write a protest to see if we can get our property, our neighbor's property and some sensitive wildlife habitat off the auction docket. As we make call after call, the common sentiment we hear from people is, *Good luck, you're fighting an uphill battle.*

We backcountry ski. We mountain bike. We know uphill.

But this mountain seems insurmountable. We are going up against the BLM, the government agency who manages the leasing of mineral rights, and the deep pockets of oil and gas companies. The cost of gas is nearing an unprecedented $4.00/gallon, accelerating this modern-day gold rush in the West.

Our anger and righteous indignation rise with the sun and never really set. The thought that our off-the-grid love nest, powered by wind and solar energy could be surrounded by oil and gas wells has turned our lovers into fighters. We are in battle, side by side with our modern weaponry of cell phones, laptops and the Internet.

He researches. I write. We work feverishly on letters of protest, letters to our congressmen, letters to the local paper trying to educate the mostly Republican ranching community that the short-term economic gains of all this aren't worth giving up the priceless beauty of our landscape and wildlife. My activist talks to a die-hard

Republican commissioner from Pinedale, Wyoming, who admits he would gladly give all the money back, if he could turn back the clock on the rampant oil and gas development his community welcomed and now regrets.

As we work side by side I see that we're not just good in bed, we are good out of it. The passion we have for each other has been directed towards saving our land and our way of life. We climb in bed at night, exhausted, but our thoughts continue to churn, processing information about surface rights, drilling rights, protest procedure. We haven't slept more than five hours a night in the past three days.

I've been on the phone so much my ear hurts. I've re-written the same paragraph five times and it still lacks conviction. I close my laptop and slide it across the kitchen table like a plate of food I'm too full to finish. I can't do anymore today.

I grab a cooler out of the shed and throw in the contents of our nearly empty fridge: elk burger, carrots, a bagel, a couple bottles of PBR and a bottle of champagne.

My activist hears me and comes out of the office. His hair is standing straight up on his head. He is wearing the same T-shirt as yesterday. I've never seen his eyes so red.

"We are going to the cabin for the night," I say. "We need a break from all this."

He stares and blinks once.

"Shower." I throw a towel at his chest and he catches it. "We can take the laptops and write there tomorrow. There isn't anyone we can call on a Sunday, anyway. We are leaving in twenty minutes."

Surprisingly, he doesn't say a word, turns and goes.

We drive the thirty miles to the cabin in silence. Both of us, I know, are visualizing oil pumps marring the canvas of our county like the ones that now dominant the landscape around Rifle, Colorado, and the Piceance Basin that contains huge reserves of natural gas. When we get to the cabin, the evening summer sun is warming the deck. I pull out two lawn chairs and the bottle of champagne, even though we have absolutely nothing to celebrate.

"We need to shift gears, have some fun, have some sex," I say as I hand him a glass. We sip in exhausted silence. We are trying hard not to talk about it all. It leaves us with nothing to say.

When I go inside to refill our glasses, I change into my favorite blue lace lingerie mini-dress. I grab his vintage brown and gold Hawaiian shirt, a hand-me-down from my dad who bought it on the big island in 1968. I throw it on his lap when I return with his champagne. He puts it on, pulls off his shorts and gets down to some zebra print Mansilk boxer briefs.

He holds his hands out to the side. "What do you think?"

We laugh. The bizarre clash of patterns and colors matches our mental distortion.

"It's perfect," I say.

We force ourselves to talk about something else: friends, kayaking, some of the clients he left behind at the kayak school. When he goes inside for another refill, he puts on the Rolling Stones. He comes out with his bottom lip rolled over and thick, like Mick's, and we end up dancing on the deck to *Shattered*. The champagne bottle is empty, our voices full, by the time we belt out, *You took my joy, I want it back* with Lucinda Williams.

I thought if we dressed up and had a party, our lovers might show up. But they don't.

My activist starts attacking the thistle in the yard with a Pulaski and then goes after the yellow jackets that have taken up residence under the eaves. Battles he can win. I slip inside the cabin and do yoga. I find myself in cobra pose with tears streaming down my face. As I lift up and back into downward dog, I exhale hard, trying to expel the ache in my shoulders, the ache in my heart. I end up weeping quietly in child's pose.

We dine on canned corn and elk burgers, leave the dishes and crawl up into the loft. We toss and turn past midnight, both of us imagining a drilling rig in the wildflower meadow outside the window.

When I awake, our bodies are already intertwined. We've reached for each other from minds that are too exhausted to think or fall into familiar lovemaking patterns. We are twisted and contorted, legs splayed, backs arched.

I find myself in a kneeling warrior position, lunging diagonally across his pelvis as I penetrate my sex with his rod. The position of my bent legs thrusting above him is ironically like a drilling rig. And that is how I feel. I am pumping him, deep, small-range thrusts that drive my clit into his pubic bone. The angle of my rig against his cock is hitting my G-spot just right, making it itch and burn. I extract my pleasure, with no sense of his, mining his body for that potent cream. My orgasm starts rising towards my throat, turning my bones to water. About now is when he usually grabs my hips and intensifies the rhythm I desperately want but don't have the strength to maintain.

But this isn't about us.

Instead, he lifts his left hip in an attempt to roll us, to take his turn. I resist and keep him pinned beneath me. There is a moment when I feel powerful, victorious and the ecstasy of it drives my orgasm straight through my larynx. I cry out just as his warrior rises up and topples mine. I am instantly flat on my back and he is above me, drilling me, thrusting fast and hard into my molten core. He takes what he wants, what he needs.

He rolls off of me. We lie panting beside each other and staring up at the ceiling. The stars outside our window are taking their leave, making room for the dawn.

"Do you have the addresses for the Congressmen on your computer?" I ask.

"Yes, I'm going to cut and paste them into the letter and do a final edit. How's the article for the paper?"

"Almost done. Another hour or so and I'll have something for you to read."

We roll towards opposite sides of the bed, get up and dress for battle.

In the end, the pool of resources we gathered with our neighbors could not begin to compete with the deep pockets of the oil and gas companies and our mineral rights sold to the highest bidder.

All we can do now is cross our fingers and hope like hell there isn't anything under there.

CHAPTER TEN

October 2006
Rule #11

I'M SURE THIS JOKE has been circulating around bachelor parties for years, but the first time I heard it was when my fiancé and I were flipping through the pages of our wedding to-do list.

"Hey, did you hear that they've discovered a food that takes away a woman's sex drive?" he asked.

"Really?" I located the notes on the reception. The only caterer in our isolated mountain community was a humorless woman who acted a lot like the old goats she tended around her double-wide. I decided that organizing the catering was now officially a groom duty.

"Please don't say chocolate."

"Wedding cake."

The line definitely delivered a punch. "Very funny," I lied.

"But you know, there's an element of truth to it."

I looked across the table at my lover and saw a flicker of fear in his eyes, something I rarely saw on the handsome, rugged face of my whitewater kayaker. But before we met, we'd both done that pick-your-opposite thing and spent years with hard-working realists, who were fine with sex once a week (or not) on Saturday mornings. We were both terrified that we could unconsciously repeat the pattern and wind up in another passionless relationship.

"Don't even talk like that," I said, a little wounded. "Besides," I continued, trying to lighten up, "we have nothing to worry about. We've never broken the loo rule."

He laughed at my reference to an article we read while traveling in New Zealand. I hadn't been able to resist buying the Kiwi's version of *Cosmo* with the cover article entitled, "Ten Rules For Avoiding a Sexless Marriage." The article seemed appropriate at the time since he had just proposed two days earlier.

Initially, we had laughed out loud when we read Rule #8: *Never use the loo in front of each other.*

But we recognized the wisdom in the advice and so far, we've honored it. "No sexless marriage!" he chants as he pushes me, toothbrush in hand, out of the bathroom.

As if he was paddling out of an eddy above a Class V rapid, my fiancé reached out and snatched the Mean Goat Lady's number. "You're right." He sounded unconvinced but fearless nonetheless. "The loo rule will save us." He picked up the phone and dialed.

I located my notes for the local women's club that I had commissioned to bake for the dessert table. *Anything chocolate* I'd written. Below it I added *No Cake* and underlined it twice.

I wasn't taking any chances.

* * *

We are on our honeymoon. For the third time. Not that we didn't get it right the first two times. On the contrary, eight days rafting the Green River in Utah in our two-person raft was gloriously right. We paddled through Class II water and red stone canyons under a warm September sun during the day. Afternoons, we lounged naked in beach camps: skinny dipping, sipping champagne and sucking fresh mango pulp off each other's non-bronzed body parts. By day six of our first honeymoon, we concluded that it would be sexual suicide to get the most romantic, passionate vacation of our marriage over with right from the start.

So we added Rule #11 to the list: *Take a honeymoon down the Green River every year.*

So here we are on day four of Honeymoon Three and we haven't had sex yet.

The only thing my legs have straddled is the black rubber pontoon of our raft as we paddle into cold headwinds. Our launch date got pushed out until early October this year because one of us was dead set on deer hunting. There are more reds and oranges in the shrub oaks hugging the banks; more yellow in the cottonwood trees that rim our beach camps. For the first time, we are experiencing snow and bloodless white toes in our Chacos. We do have the river to ourselves (imagine that!), which is ultimately romantic to us. We could have sex anywhere we wanted if it would just get warm enough to take off our clothes, which hasn't happened yet.

We're dressed more for skiing than desert rafting as we break camp and launch into the icy dawn. The string bikini I wear beneath the layers of polypropylene, fleece and Gortex defines optimism. We haven't seen each other's bodies in four days, which is such a shame since we've been paddling our asses off and thus buffing out our pecs, lats and biceps.

We move in silence as we synchronize our paddle strokes in an effort to get warm. The trill of a canyon wren floats out to us from the riverbank. Usually the call feels like a melodious caress from the canyon, but this morning it sounds like a heckle. Our insuppressible moans are the only other sounds as we work the lactic acid out of our aching muscles. The tension we are feeling, however, isn't just between our shoulder blades.

In the weeks leading up to this trip we'd been having... shall we say….a less-sex marriage. There was a cold, a cold sore, menstruation. My husband juggled raft guiding, hunting, and finishing his thesis for his master's degree in wildlife biology. I overbooked myself with yoga classes and a race against the onset of winter to finish an outdoor painting project at my studio. We abused caffeine and slept little knowing we would be rewarded with a honeymoon at the finish line.

But the finish line has yet to appear. Scraping the ancient wood trim of the 'historic' building that houses my yoga studio sounds like a piece of cake (by no means the wedding cake variety) compared to the last three days of this trip.

After four years of outdoor adventures with this man, I've learned when exhaustion has barbed my tongue and it is best not to speak. This is definitely one of those times.

"The good news is we're almost done with the flat water," he says. After four years of taking me down rivers and avalanche chutes, he can tell when I am about to crack. "We'll be coming into some rapids today and should make Lion Hollow camp by dinner." In our guidebook, we have three stars by Lion Hollow, which was the site of Mexican night on Honeymoon #2 when we sucked little tequila shots from each other's navels before launching into an oral sex contest.

What I say: "That sounds good."

What I don't say: *What do you mean the good news? There is no good news. We are doomed like all the other foolish romantics who dare to get married. We're having a sexless marriage. Kiwi Cosmo lied.*

"We can't do anything about the weather," he continues, "but I have a feeling this storm is moving out today."

What I say: "Oh, I hope so."

What I don't say: *We wouldn't be in this storm if we had kept our original September launch date. Why the hell did we postpone our trip for deer hunting? Is this inevitable in a marriage, a freezer full of wild game takes precedence over a romantic river trip? The honeymoons are over.*

"At least we aren't working."

I can't even think of a benign response to that one because right now my cozy yoga studio sounds heavenly. I start paddling harder in an attempt to move into my body and away from my head and its negative, over-analyzing psyche. But it is relentless: *Maybe there is a magic inherent in firsts—the first kiss, the first fuck, the first honeymoon—that you just can't recreate. We just got lucky with Honeymoon #2. We got greedy by going for a third. We've set ourselves up for disappointment and even worse, created that which we fear the most.*

I know this line of thinking isn't productive, so I try to focus on a simple achievable goal: paddling until our mid-morning coffee break. The thermos of coffee is our greatest source of pleasure right now, a tough reality for a couple of hedonists who expected a week of sun-filled debauchery and sex. But as the morning progresses, the gray clouds start to break exposing a sky that is getting bluer with every paddle stroke.

By the time we pull out the thermos, we lose the fleece gloves and exchange the ski hats for baseball caps. By lunch, we are shedding like snakes, ditching the Gortex pants, jackets and fleece. Our spirits rise like warm air currents as we hit rapids the color and temperature of an iced latte in shorts and long sleeved T-shirts. I've been taking the crashing waves between my thighs, savoring the alternately numbing and tingling sensations of the icy river water on my clit. Between rapids, the sun warms the black rubber pontoon between my thighs. I tilt my pelvis forward and let its warmth permeate my cold cunt.

With rapids and no headwinds, we make Lion Hollow by late afternoon and the blessed yellow sun is still hovering overhead. I don't know who names these river campsites, but unlike the river itself (the Green River is the brownest river I've ever paddled), this site was properly named. A pride of lions belongs here, lounging about in the various hollows of sand tucked amidst yellowing cottonwoods, tamarisk and juniper.

Normally, we get our chores done first: unload the raft and organize camp. There is no need to discuss our break from protocol. I strip down to my bikini as soon as my foot hits the shore. My husband is already digging through the cooler making rum and pineapple juice cocktails. I grab the picnic blanket from our waterproof lunch bucket.

My legs feel as rubbery as our raft as we trudge up the dunes in search of a place for our long-awaited beach party. We spread our blanket at the first flat sunny spot, take a few sips of our drinks and lie back, eager to finally feel the warmth of the desert sun on our skin. The heat of it is like a balm on our sore muscles and as sweet as the rum pineapple juice that dribbles down our necks as we try unsuccessfully to drink while lying down.

I want to capture the bliss of this moment, but of course the camera is buried in a dry bag strapped to the boat.

"Click," I say. My husband's hand reaches over to mine and begins to stroke my wrist. Mine floats over and caresses his thigh.

And then in the cruelest of jokes yet from this desert sky, the sun disappears. Even though it is still hovering in the sky, it has dropped behind a tall, red stone mesa that frames this campsite to the west. I wonder if the sky is conspiring against us.

"Nooooo!" I scream and curl up like a caterpillar. Not one to be defeated, my husband jumps to his feet looking for options.

"Come on," he says as he grabs my hand and pulls me up. "We just have to hike higher up the dune. The sun is still up there."

He grabs the drinks. I drag the blanket as we hike uphill through the sand. My legs are burning with fatigue, so after five minutes of climbing and sipping we call it good and plop back down on the blanket.

I extend my legs and stretch forward to release the ache in my lower back. My husband does the same. As I spread my legs and lean to one side, I feel the sun warming my sex as my husband's hand reaches over and caresses the expanse of my ribcage. The warmth of their mutual touch, two sensations I've been craving for days, makes me shiver with pleasure. As I stretch to the other side, I reach over and caress his thigh, letting my hand drift across the growing bulge in his shorts. We stretch and touch, marveling in the sight and feel of each other's skin. Our bodies are gifts to be unwrapped. I discover striated pecs in his chest, and hard lats that funnel down to his waist where my hand slides beneath his shorts. I push his shorts down his legs as I stretch forward. His hand brushes over my ripe sex, tugs at one of the bows of my bikini bottom and releases it.

He pushes the small triangle of fabric away and begins stroking my outer lips as my mouth moves forward to kiss the smooth head of his erection. My folds are starting to melt like warm wax, but then my flesh contracts in protest as the sun drops once again behind the mesa.

There is a litany of cursing but no hesitation this time, both of us knowing what we must do. My husband drags our blanket behind him as his erection points up hill to the highest point on the dune that is still bathed in yellow light. My bikini bottoms hang by one bow as I scoop up our cocktails. Our blood pumps with lust and rum as we run through the deep sand. We are laughing, panting and parched when we get to the top. We finish the cocktails and toss the plastic cups to the side.

He tugs at the other bow at my hip, releasing my dangling bikini. I fall to my knees on the blanket and reach for his cock. He pulls at the bows at my back and neck freeing my breasts before diving between my legs.

Although we haven't bathed in four days, we are clean where it counts. The French have bidets. Rafters have crotch shots in the rapids.

We launch into 69, simultaneously sucking on each other knowing that we don't have much time. I kiss and flick my tongue.

He does the same. When he sucks my clit deeply, rhythmically between his lips, I mimic, sliding him in and out of my throat. I am already starting to quiver as he pulls his hips back from my face. After four days of drudgery, we are both struggling to breathe from the intensity of giving and receiving so much pleasure. We sit up and our faces meet, our tongues tangling and devouring the tastes of each other. I lie back pulling him on top of me.

His body is hot from the desert sun and this passion that has finally been kindled. He rubs the head of his cock against my clit in a quick tease before sliding in. My sex has been cold and wet for days and the warmth of his sun-drenched cock melting into me sends my sheath into spasms of ecstasy. I am suddenly reminded of our tantric sex book and its referral to the penis as a lingam or 'wand of light'. At the time, giving his cock some New Age name seemed really hokey, but right now, it is so fucking right on. He is lighting me up, radiating heat within my cold, contracted core so that it liquefies and gushes with each thrust.

I roll us to the side desperate for a view. Each time he emerges from my fuzzier than usual peach, his wand, slick from my juices, indeed glistens in the desert sunlight. We undulate slowly, both of us mesmerized by the visual of this long-awaited communion.

I want to feel him every way so I roll to my belly. When he mounts me from behind, his four-day beard tickles my neck prompting a shiver that streaks down my spine like a shooting star. When it collides at my cervix with the pumping heat of his wand, my sheath starts to quake. He knows to give me more. A low growl emerges from his throat as he continues to nuzzle and thrust. We are positioned on our hands and knees, mating like the wild cats this camp is named for. Like them, we are ravenous for warm flesh. My arm reaches back and claws his haunches. When he bites me on the shoulder, I feel it radiate down to my clit like a lightning bolt.

I buck back into him wanting that hard lingam cock as deep as it can go. His sack spanks up against me, the sound of flesh on flesh, a primal percussive.

He pauses.

"Don't stop," I beg.

"I won't last."

"Neither will the sun." We are at the highest point on the dune looking over the river; there is nowhere else to run to chase the sun's warmth.

He grabs my cheeks with both hands and the exquisite burn floods my sheath as he continues to thrust. 'Wand' is suddenly too tame a term for this rocket combusting inside of me. When he comes, we shudder from the blast that raises our bodies and propels us up onto our knees. I wrap my arms back around his neck, as his hands play me like a stand-up bass, one hand strumming a nipple while the other fingers my clit, working me up to one final crescendo as the last rays of sun leave our bodies.

We fall forward and I land on my belly. The weight and heat of him warms me like a blanket. We are laughing, spent and getting cooler by the second. We need to make a move.

"Are you ready?" he whispers in my ear.

I can guess what he is thinking: that he wants me to keep our connection tight as I lift up and back for a simultaneous downward dog pose so our juices saturate the sand instead of our blanket. It's a move we perfected on Honeymoon #1.

"Downward Dog?"

"Yeah, but then we are going to get up and run down the dunes and without stopping, without hesitating, we are going to dive right into the river."

I can't think of anything I'd rather do less.

"Okay," I hear myself say.

I feel the heat of his breath on my ear. "Three...two...one...blastoff!"

We push back into downward dog. The desert air slaps at my dripping entrance as my rocket man pulls away and starts running. I cross my arms beneath my breasts for support and chase him down the shaded dune as the warmth of our ecstasy trickles down my inner thigh.

By the time we get back down to the river I am freezing and losing my nerve. My husband doesn't hesitate for a second, doesn't miss a step. I watch his torso and then his haunches disappear into the brown river. Like it has been these past four years with this adventurer of mine, I swallow my reservations, tighten my jaw and dive.

We both emerge, laughing, panting and trying to find our breath. The cooling desert air feels warm now in comparison to the numbing river water. I splash between my legs and feel an aftershock tremor in my clit.

"Turn around," he says.

"Why?"

"No sexless marriage," he explains as he hugs himself for warmth. If we were home right now, he'd be pushing me and my toothbrush towards the door.

I throw my arms out, opening my chest to the desert dusk in one of those victorious, crossing-the-finish-line postures.

"No Sexless Marriage!" I shout. My voice travels down the river as it echoes off the canyons walls.

We must look like a couple of crazed natives, standing naked in the brown river, laughing and splashing as we take turns shouting our mantra.

We revel in the sound of the desert chanting it back to us.

CHAPTER ELEVEN

January 2007
Yang My Yin

FROM MY NEST ON THE COUCH, I watch the sinewy muscles of my man's bare back twitch as he stands in front of the sliding glass door of our cabin, a pair of binoculars glued to his face. His torso triangulates, funneling into the waistband of his silk boxer briefs, much like the avalanche chute he is viewing on Mount Hailey. Outside it is snowing lightly, a small break in the storm that's been predicted to dump another foot of champagne powder. Inside we're barely dressed, seduced down to our underwear from the heat of the wood-burning stove.

"I can hardly see our tracks from yesterday," he says. I hear the next thought that he doesn't speak. *We should have been out there today, carving it up again.*

I moan and sink deeper into the soft cushions of our chenille couch. We've spent the last three weeks gorging on the record-breaking snow, skiing the backcountry during the coldest, darkest days of a Rocky Mountain winter. Every cell of my being is exhausted. The words *athletic* and *adventurous* aren't in my vocabulary today. I lost them yesterday when after five hours of climbing up and skiing down Mount Hailey, we buried our snowmobile in a monstrous drift on the way back to the cabin.

"I want to be boring!" My voice echoed in the woods that were suddenly rendered silent when our snowmobile choked and died on three feet of snow. My skier laughed as he pulled our avalanche shovels from our ski packs.

"Hey, I got an idea." He barely suppressed a grin as he handed me my shovel. "We could go golfing."

He's mastered the art of making me laugh when I'm so tired I want to cry. My previous boyfriend wanted me to take up golfing with him. Horrified, I lobbied hard for more mountain biking. The nail in the coffin to our dying relationship was when he gave me a pair of golfing shoes for my birthday.

"Touché," I said as I grabbed the shovel.

"Tomorrow," he stepped forward and sank up to his crotch in snow, "you can be boring."

"Promise?" I asked.

He didn't answer. Instead he gave me a feigned hurt look that conveyed: *You doubt me?*

Yes, I doubted him. The man never tires. He would have climbed Mount Hailey again today, but with the avalanche conditions as they are, it would have been dangerous for him to go alone. (I think it's dangerous that he believes I would have the presence of mind to track his buried body with my avalanche beacon and dig him out without completely freaking out, but that is a different story.)

So today, I've been burrowing into the couch trying to hide from the guilt of making us miss such an amazing powder day. My tomboy persona hasn't been helping.

"Cowboy up, slug," she taunts, towering above me on the couch with her hands on her polypropylene encased hips. I thought I'd left her behind on a mogul slope when I was twenty–five, but when my skier stepped into the scene five years ago she came charging back to center stage. Her messy braids sprout in every direction, creating a haphazard frame of blonde around her chapped red cheeks. I've been letting her have free rein lately and she's become demanding and spoiled.

"Go away," I tell her as I nestle under my quilt. "Wash your hair." I've managed to keep up with her the past week by downing energy bars and thick black tea from my stainless steel thermos. But I have absolutely nothing to give her today. I gave what little I had left to that snowdrift last night.

My skier is still at the sliding glass door. He gives me the snow report on the east face of the mountain now, convinced that the lower-angled slope there will be safe to ski tomorrow. The muscle twitch has settled into his left buttock that looks so round and hard that I imagine myself slithering off the couch and across the wood floors to bite it. But even though I've been reading and napping all day, that simple act of lust feels too ambitious.

It's not fair. My man never needs a day on the couch. He doesn't have a cyclical rhythm, just one steady uphill pulse. His maleness has been pacing around the cabin all day like a caged panther. My femininity has been burrowing into the couch like a mole. We are both in extreme states of our gender archetype.

He is yang, like the sun, that never burns dim.

I am yin, like the moon, that waxes and wanes. I feel the moon's pull on my body as I rub my hands over my heavy uterus.

Somewhere between the two of us there is a balance. I beckon him to the couch in an attempt to find it.

"Give me some of that," I say as I reach for him.

He is puzzled at first, since usually it's his food that I am after and he isn't eating any.

"Some of what?" he asks, displaying his empty hands. I pull his hips to my face and nuzzle my nose into his briefs.

"Some of this," I say as I cup his silky package in my hands.

His hands come to rest on my head as he caresses my hair.

"Take," he says as he exhales long and slow, "whatever you want."

I rub my face against the silky fabric enjoying the feel of it against my weathered skin. As he springs to arousal, I peel away the silk, craving that hard maleness of him. I wrap my lips around his tip, inviting him into the dark cave of my mouth with my tongue. He has so much of what I need. I pull him deep into my throat and swallow, ingesting it.

His hands drift to my neck where he gently rubs the kink that has been plaguing me all week from skiing up steep mountain faces with a heavy gear-filled pack. His caress drops to my breasts that are tender now, like ripe peaches. He cradles them, letting his thumbs whisper across my nipples, making them hard.

In yin/yang theory, the opposing energies in the universe are complimentary, each containing a seed of the other. We are watering each other's.

I feel his pulse in my throat and it enlivens mine. My hands that were too tired to open a jar of salsa at breakfast are suddenly recharged and eager to explore. One teases and tickles his testicles while the other encircles the base of his shaft. I am milking him with palm, lips and tongue, thirsty for the vitality that infuses his cream. He moans and pulls away, wanting to prolong our ecstasy but I will not allow it. I'm not after a long multi-orgasmic experience here.

You've heard of medicinal marijuana. Well, this is a medicinal fuck.

I'm already feeling stronger as I grab his hips and turn, forcing him to sit on the couch. This is the most energy I've had all day and I want more. I mount him, lowering the deepest, most yin part of my body onto the hard yang of his erection, initiating the ultimate balance of opposites. I intentionally squeeze and contract around him as I thrust, desperate now to feel his potent essence explode inside my core.

A voice inside my head chants in rhythm with my thrusts like some transcending priestess. *Infuse me, infuse me, infuse me…*

He knows that I want it now, that I want it fast and he doesn't hold back. He grabs the flesh of my butt and pushes even deeper into me, driving my clit into his pubic bone. My sheath responds in spasmodic contractions as he releases inside me. I've read my tantra, and imagine my orgasm drawing his vitality up the entire length of my body, alighting my chakras in the colors of the spectrum as it rises to my crown and bursts in a fountain of iridescent white light that floats down around me like the powdery snow outside our window.

He relaxes inside me, lured into the dark, restful place there. We close our eyes, savoring the exchange.

I notice the quiet rhythm of his breathing and realize he has drifted off to sleep while still embraced within my body. His eyes flutter as I guide him down into my nest on the couch. Sliding off him, I notice a pink tinge to our fluids as I wipe them away. I pull the quilt up to his chin, kiss his forehead and leave him to succumb to the yin. Teeming now with yang, I tiptoe away.

Outside the sliding glass door, the sky to the west has become a magnificent battleground between the fiery setting sun and the next wave of dark, ominous storm clouds. Energized, I pull on fleece,

Gortex and snow shoes, eager to witness the sun's last exertion for the day before the storm claims victory.

As I stomp towards the sunset through sagebrush white and rounded with snow, I sense something behind me. When I look over my shoulder, I am stunned by the beauty of the moon rising up in the east, huge and round from behind Ute Peak. The skies this month have been so dense with snow clouds that I haven't seen her in weeks. She is waxing and full like me.

The orange and magenta light of the setting sun swirls across the sky towards the full moon and reminds me of the Chinese symbol for yin and yang: the white swirling into the black.

I imagine my man's white ejaculate swirling within the dark crimson of my uterus, bringing me back to balance.

CHAPTER TWELVE

February 2007
First Time

THE FEBRUARY MORNING is so cold, dawn can barely break outside our loft window. My breath hovers, cloudlike, in front of my face so I burrow under the covers until I find the curve and heat of my lover's haunches. I piggy back up to his warmth and flatten my breasts and belly against his back. When I wrap my arm around his ribcage, he grabs my hand and pulls it to his chest.

The thermometer had already dipped way below zero last night when we arrived by snowmobile to our frozen cabin. Even though we fed the woodstove for three hours, the olive oil on the kitchen shelf was still solid when we climbed into bed under a mound of wool and down blankets. We lost the fire around midnight and soon after I felt my husband add the weight of an elk hide to our nest. The forecast predicted a low of minus thirty degrees.

I can barely hear my husband's voice from beneath the covers, but I know what he is saying.

"Coffee."

I nuzzle up to his ear and kiss him. "I got it yesterday morning."

"I got it two mornings in a row before that."

I can't remember, but I know he is bluffing. "No way."

He rolls over to face me and positions his pillow on top of our heads for warmth.

"Best two out of three," he says as he pulls his hand from mine. "One, two, three..." I lift my hand up in a fist.

We both throw rock.

He counts to three again.

And then we both throw scissors.

"That's never happened before," I say. "What do we do now?"

Before I even finish my sentence he starts counting backwards from five.

"No!" I scream as I dive under.

"...three, two, one, blast off!" he yells as he rips the covers off our naked bodies.

This is my least favorite way for him to take my breath away.

My arms hug instinctively around my indignant nipples that are contracting so hard it hurts.

"Come on." He pries my hands from my chest and pulls me out of bed. "We're both going."

He untangles the clothes beside the bed that we peeled out of last night and tosses me my fleece tights, polypro shirt and wool sweater. We are both cursing the cold under the frigid smoke of our breath as we scramble to dress.

On mornings like this, I wonder what it would be like to be married to a regular guy, someone with a furnace, a heated garage and a driveway instead of a snowmobile trail.

Two balled-up wool socks hit me in the chest. I pull them on and scurry down the loft stairs behind my husband. He goes right to the wood stove. I head left towards the kitchen. I fill up the teakettle, grateful that the five-gallon water jug we hauled in didn't freeze overnight. The lighter is too cold to light, so I dig around until I find some matches. I set up the French press with coffee, blow on my fingers to warm them and hurry down to the woodstove that is popping and crackling to life.

"Here," he says as he holds out my down jacket for me. I slide it on and he pushes my wool ski hat on my head.

"I can't believe you did that."

"What? You look cute in your ski hat." He kisses me.

"I can't believe you ripped the covers off."

"It's like ripping off a Band-Aid, you just have to do it quick and get it over with."

"Brutal." I shiver

"Exhilarating. When it gets this cold, you just have to embrace it...and the beautiful woman standing next to you."

He grabs me and pulls me into his body. We rub against each other trying to create some friction until the teakettle whistles.

Since heat rises, the loft warms up first, so we head back up there with our coffee and climb back into bed fully dressed.

The aspen branches outside the window are fuzzy with frost. The bright blue Stellar jays at the birdfeeder look like they are pumped up on steroids. The chickadees, usually the first to the feeder, aren't even up yet.

"I remember the first time you brought me coffee in bed," I say between sips.

"Really? I can't remember that." He peels off his down jacket and slides deeper under the covers, settling in for one of his favorite stories.

"Well," I begin. "It all started when you came to my Christmas Open House at the yoga studio and invited me out to your cabin for lunch."

"You forgot the part about how you couldn't think straight during your open house because I was there and how you kept gravitating to where I was standing," he adds.

"Right, and after everyone left when I was cleaning up, I found a down coat and it was yours and I wore it the rest of the night."

"Little did I know that you were planning on seducing me the next day at my cabin," he says.

"Me, seduce you? It was the other way around."

He is quiet, trying to remember the fine details of our love affair that we both cherish like sunny October days on the Green River. My memory usually trumps his, but the truth is the assault was mutual. He brought me out to the cabin by snowmobile, the only way to access it in the winter. After a snowshoe hike up Ute Ridge we stretched in front of the woodstove in our polypro shirts and tights while we waited for rice to cook for lunch.

We'd been working under the pretense of being friends because I had a boyfriend. But when I tried to do the right thing and talk to the golfer about the attraction I had to one of my yoga students, he didn't take it very well. He made a pile of the few things I had at his house—an erotica book, a toothbrush and some tampons—and left them on the porch.

So, in all fairness, the newly single me reached out to caress the sinewy muscles of the adventurer's forearm because I'd been dying to for weeks.

"I remember now, you reached over and grabbed my cock and told me you wanted to fuck me," he says.

"I did not! I put my hand on your arm and said I wanted to *touch* you."

"Same thing. What happened next?"

"I didn't realize I was opening the door to a lion's cage when I *touched* you. Your passion came charging out and attacked me."

"The first pounce," he says. There was no first kiss for us, no slow leaning forward and connecting of the lips. As soon as my hand made contact with his forearm, the rest of our limbs followed suit. A flood of kisses warmed my neck as his hands floated up and down my body. I remember feeling overwhelmed with sensation, grabbing one of his hands and holding it over my heart that was beating so fast I could hardly breathe.

We've been doing this dance for years now in white water and avalanche chutes: he slows things down a notch and I step forward out of my comfort zone.

As new lovers do, we luxuriated in kissing, taking time to explore each other's tastes and textures until the smell of burning rice pulled us towards a bottle of wine and lunch.

As if he can hear my thoughts, he says, "That was a superior move on my part, opening the bottle of Cabernet with lunch."

"So European," I joke.

"More of an American guy, get-her-drunk tactic I'm afraid," he admits as he takes my empty coffee cup and sets it on the windowsill. He helps me slide out of my down jacket and pulls the ski hat off my head.

"And then when the wine was gone and we were getting ready to clean up and leave because you had to be at a fundraiser that night, you said..."

He recites his line brilliantly. "I'm not trying to lure you into my bedroom or anything, but you have to check this out..."

"And there was a three quarter moon rising up in the alpenglow of the sunset," I say remembering the way the rising moon hung in the pink and orange sky outside the loft window.

"Purely innocent move there, I didn't know yet that you were a lunatic."

He pulls my sweater over my head and frames my face between his hands. We are in bed, in our polypropylene underwear, the past blending so exquisitely with the present.

He kisses me, his mouth moist, watering mine. One hand cradles my head and caresses my hair. The other drops down, caressing the heat of my sex through my tights. My hand drifts across the bulge in his tights. Our hands move slowly, exploring the landscapes of each other, as if it was the first time.

I pull away his shirt revealing his muscular torso made all the more masculine by the pelt of dark hair that funnels down his hard abdomen. My touch is reverent, as if I've been granted permission to touch the statue of David. Like David, his muscles are chiseled, sculpted by his passions for white water kayaking and backcountry skiing.

He reaches for the bottom of my shirt. I am not wearing a bra but he pauses for me to recite my line anyway.

I cringe at this part, trying to summon up the playfulness I felt then when he fumbled with the clasp of my bra and I reached back to assist him.

"Are you ready to meet my breasts?" I say. He peels my shirt away exposing my breasts and cups them gently in his hands, then he dives right between my legs.

There are breast men and there are pussy men.

We laugh now the way we did back then as he peels my tights down my legs. He tucks a finger under the elastic of my panties and slides it slowly back and forth across my belly before leaning down and kissing the heat of my sex through the lace. The first time I wore a black nylon bikini—thank God I wasn't wearing the white cotton Hanes. But now I am wearing the pink lace thong he gave me for Christmas. He grabs it in his teeth and pulls it down my legs pausing to kiss my inner thighs as he descends.

I peel away his polypro tights and reach for him, remembering that first afternoon in the loft, when suddenly the man I fantasized about for weeks during yoga class kneeled before me wearing nothing but a piece of jade around his neck and the most magnificent hard-on I'd ever seen, rising out of his core like a scepter pointing to the sky.

"Your magnificent cock," I whisper because I know how much he loves to hear me say it.

I take him into my mouth, feeling as hungry for him now as I did then, his hands gently caressing my head as he moans. I savor the feel of his cock, so smooth yet so hard with just a hint of his musky arousal lingering in the fur around his testicles. I breathe in the animal scent of him and tickle his testicles with my fingertips as I suck.

And then he pulls away.

"Everything felt so good I wanted to make it last," he says as he guides me down on my back. And it wasn't just the first time that he put off his pleasure to prolong ours. Unlike any of my previous lovers, he savors my pleasure as much as his own.

His gaze locks on mine, his brown eyes still penetrating and filled with lust.

"You never close your eyes," I say my line, prompting his.

"And miss all this beauty?" he asks. I love to hear him say it. His hands and eyes caress me simultaneously. "Your pale skin, blue eyes and blonde hair strewn across the pillow..."

"You looked into my eyes the entire time."

"When I wasn't licking your sweet pussy," he says as he descends.

The golfer used to joke about doing 68: "You do me and I'll owe you one." It wasn't really a joke. So to have a man descend on me with such passion and desire launched my clit into spasms of anticipatory orgasms before his tongue even made contact. My clit buzzes from the memory. His lips land warm and moist on the flesh of my inner thigh as his hands contour the curve of my waist. His tongue moves tantalizingly slow across my vulva, tasting, savoring, exploring. He uses his lips and fingers to open my petals, exposing my swollen bud that he tickles with his flicking tongue.

I quickly learned that this man excels at everything he does including cunnilingus.

The first time, I remember pulling his face from between my thighs and kissing him, wanting to taste myself on his lips.

There was talk of a condom, but then we noticed the clock.

"You had other plans that night because you really thought we would just have lunch..." I continue the story of our first sexual encounter.

"...I had no idea that a goddess like you would be interested in a guy like me."

"Goddesses love lions," I say, amazed still at his humility. "Time had evaporated and it was well into evening and you were late. Part of me wanted you to ignore your commitment but I was so impressed when you didn't."

"People were expecting me."

"So we stopped, not wanting to rush through the next part. No penetration, no intercourse," I say as I stroke the dark hair of his pelt. "We rushed around pulling on clothes, tucking away dirty dishes and then we jumped on the snowmobile and took off into the starry night."

"We saw a falling star," he says.

"I whispered in your ear to make a wish." I kiss his ear. "And you said..."

"My wish just came true." I feel tears pool in my eyes like the first time he said it. And I realize, as I always do, that I don't need a heated garage or a furnace or a driveway.

I just need this man.

CHAPTER THIRTEEN

May 2007
Parting Shots

REMEMBER THIS, **SHE THINKS:** The California morning sun on his face. His eyes, the lids still heavy with sleep, tracking her as she saunters across the flattened grass of their isolated riverside camp. His hair, dark and messy with sleep, splayed against the maroon flannel of his pillowcase. His smile when he notices the small bottle in her hand, like a boy about to get an ice cream cone on a hot summer day.

She matches his smile with her own as she slowly unscrews the lid, both of them knowing he is about to get an adult male's equivalent of a triple scoop.

Remember this, he thinks: The dusting of freckles along her shoulders as she lays her body perpendicular to his, her nose flirting with his growing erection. The cool stickiness of her touch as she finger-paints his rod and sack with Grand Marnier. The seductive smile on her face as she takes a sip, slithers up his body and kisses him. The singe of the liqueur as it vaporizes up his sinuses. The velvet swath of her tongue as she descends, licking him in long, slow strokes. Her eyes, the color of the sky, rolling back beneath fluttering lids as she slides him deep into her throat. The exquisite burn of her hands beneath him, squeezing his cheeks as she pulses him in and out.

Remember this, she thinks: The way his hand reaches down and burrows between her thighs when she sucks him from the side like this. The sound of his low, gravely moans, making her sheath salivate like one of Pavlov's dogs. The flutter of his fingers against her labia, a teasing rap at her entrance, as if he needs permission to enter.

She pushes herself into the palm of his hand, circling her hips as she circles her tongue around his tip. As his fingers spiral in on her clitoris, she pauses, savoring. *Store this*, she thinks, so when she wakes up without him in the month to come, her own touch will make her clit quiver like this, like the wings of a hummingbird.

Remember this, he thinks: The spread of her thighs across his hips, her strawberry blond strip penetrating his dark curls. Their scent rising between them, a heady blend of sex, earth, and orange liqueur. The downward pressure of her palms against his chest as she thrusts and grinds with her entire being. The flush rising up her throat that escapes in a gasp as he grabs her hips, intensifying their rhythm. *Keep this*, he thinks, so when he wakes alone to the cry of osprey and the urge of his morning wood, he can imagine the slick heat of her core contracting all around him, wanting him deeper and deeper until he explodes.

Remember this, she thinks: The satiety on his face, the ooze of their ecstasy warm and slippery between them. His hands lifting, forming a box, pushing the imaginary shutter release with his index finger. *Click*, he says and she realizes he's been doing it too, trying to sear this morning into memory. Their digital camera has been buried somewhere in the truck and they haven't taken a single picture all week, probably the only people to visit Yosemite who could claim that. But no photograph could capture this anyway: this moment, so pure, so alive, like the river beside them bursting with spring.

Remember this, he thinks: The sun like a halo behind her head, her blond hair cascading over her breasts like spun gold. He holds up his hands, trying to frame her in his memory. *Click*, he says. He watches her beam even brighter from his adoration, sweeping her arms overhead, lifting her breasts, fanning her lats, posing for him in a way she would be too shy to do if the camera was real. She gives him a sly, downward look, her hair sliding across one eye, a shimmering veil. *Yes*, he thinks. *Click. Click.*

Remember this, she thinks as she looks up from packing and searching her duffle bag for something clean to wear on the plane. The grace of his movement as he pulls away his shorts and lets them drop from his fingers as if they never belonged there in the first place. His carved buttocks, concaved at the sides and white like alabaster, between the bronzed flesh of his torso and legs. The half-smile of his profile as he looks over his shoulder, enticing her down to the river. The precision of his barefoot steps, down the rocky hillside as he drops from sight into the smoke-colored white water.

Remember this, he thinks as he stands above her on a rock and towels himself dry. The supple bend to her spine, the compact strength of her muscles as she arches backward to let the river rinse her hair. The sun dancing all over her body, refracting off the diamond stud in her belly button, shimmering in the river water that clings to her contracted nipple.

He watches his two greatest passions, his wife and the river, completely enthralled with each other. *Click.*

Remember this, she thinks: The icy thrill of current sliding across her travel-weary body that is sticky with sunscreen, sweat and sex. The ache of the river's cold nimble fingers across her scalp, through her hair, as she leans back and lowers her head under a small waterfall.

She gasps, laughs and turns, moving her pubis into the flow, rinsing away their juices, willing the ones inside to absorb into her core as it contracts from the chill. *Stay,* she thinks, wanting to feel him seep out of her somewhere over Nevada. Her clit tingles as she cups water in her hands and splashes herself. *Goodbye river, be sweet to my kayaker.* She scoops up another handful of the river and tosses it up toward the sun, letting it shower down on her in rainbows.

Remember this, he thinks, as he reaches for her hand across the console as they near the San Francisco airport. We may not always have this longing before we part, these strong youthful bodies, the gift of this potent love. As he embraces her by the departures curb, he buries his face in her hair, smelling lichen and warm gray rock.

Remember this, she thinks as she watches the earth drop away outside her window. She reaches for her notebook and begins to write, photographing the morning with her words, framing it for him.

*   *   *

She is spooned behind him, caressing his back the way she does when she is awake and wanting him to be as well. He summons a moan of encouragement and her hand descends, circling around the hard curve of his buttock before sliding down the back of his thigh. She nudges his top leg forward with hers and cups his testicles in her palm, letting her fingers lightly drum against the base of his shaft. His cock twitches. She grasps him fully as her lips nuzzle his neck. She kisses him, her tongue wet, too wet, licking the side of his face. He opens his eyes to see the snout of the kayak school's blue heeler.

"Mazie," he says with a disappointed sigh. He grabs the dog's head and pulls her down on his sleeping bag. He rubs her neck as he turns to avoid her lapping tongue. The sun is already burning away the coastal fog that shrouds the river at night and as his head clears, he vaguely remembers turning off the alarm on his watch. He checks the time, realizes he's overslept and jumps out of his sleeping bag, urging his hard-on into his Gramicci pants. He knows from experience that it will be gone by the time he gets up to the lodge for a cup of coffee.

As he walks past the kayak school's organic garden, he sees the owner of the lodge, his boss, pulling weeds, already two hours into his workday. "I sent Mazie down to wake you up," he says with a smirk. "I see it worked."

"Send a curvaceous blond next time." He runs a hand through his messy dark hair.

"Speaking of which, there is a letter in there for you. I propped it next to the coffee pot."

"Coffee," he mumbles, but his steps are lighter, faster now. Inside, he pours himself a cup and takes the envelope addressed to him in her unmistakable script of all capital letters that don't quite finish themselves. He is about to open it when one of the guests approaches him with a question about their kayak roll. He is suddenly holding court with a group of students: two lawyers, a neurosurgeon, and a retired general, who are all excited about their first day of paddling on moving water. Some egos will drown. He tucks the envelope into his pocket, so he can savor her letter when he is alone.

*   *   *

She wakes up as dawn is breaking the Colorado sky into shards of pink and orange and pulls his pillow close to her chest. After three weeks, his scent is dwindling but she can still detect a trace of his head-hair scent lingering on the pillowcase. She looks at the clock and knows he still sleeps on his beach beside the Salmon River. She lets her hand flow up and down the pillow as if it was his back, caressing him awake like she loves to do.

She reaches around her pillow, all the way to California and lets her fingers float around the soft flesh of his unsuspecting package. She wraps her palm around his sleepy cock, imagining it twitching and expanding in her grasp. She presses her lips against his neck and hears a low reverberating sound, one of his moans encouraging her. She hears it again, louder this time, like a gong, and realizes it's coming from outside her window. Her curiosity pulls her from her fantasy. When she looks outside, she half-expects to see a Tibetan monk sitting beneath the aspen summoning her to meditation.

Instead, she sees a male grouse trying desperately to get laid. He is working it hard, spreading his elaborate plumage, expanding his chest and pumping his throat, releasing the gong sound that she assumes is some kind of mating call. She sees movement in the sage and can barely detect a female grouse scurrying away in a flurry of brown feathers. She jumps out of bed, and follows from window to window until the female grouse flies across the meadow with the male in hot pursuit. She ends up at her computer, as she often does, channeling her lust into her keyboard.

* * *

Ten hours later when the guests are having appetizers and wine at the lodge, he pulls out her letter. He is sitting by the river, wet from a swim, a cold beer on the sand beside him. He's been waiting all day for a chance to be alone with her words. On top of the fourteen-hour workdays, there is no internet or cell phone coverage at the remote kayak school, so they haven't been able to communicate much at all in the past three weeks. He runs his fingers over her name in the upper left corner of the envelope before tearing it open.

He hears voices coming down the trail, two of the other kayak instructors, and tunes them out as he begins to read. But he quickly realizes that she didn't send a letter after all, but one of her stories. He gets to the second paragraph and knows he can't read it now, feeling already how hard it's going to make him. He tucks it back into its envelope and pulls a towel over his lap as he watches his co-workers strip off their clothes and dive into the river.

Even though he skips the chocolate mousse and port, he isn't able to extract himself from dinner until after ten o'clock. The full moon is so bright he doesn't even need his headlamp as he makes his way down to the beach. He throws his sleeping bag down on the sand and pulls out her story. Although the white computer paper glows in the moonlight, he switches on his headlamp to read the black type.

Her words transport him back to the Tuolumne River on their last morning together. Her blonde hair strewn across his belly, the freckled tip of her nose nudging his cock which expands in his hand with every word he reads.

Remember this, she writes and he does. And then some. His grip on his cock tightens as he remembers the clenching of her throat all around him when she pulls him so deep that it makes her gag. The flicking of her tongue, light as raindrops, around his balls as she works him with her hand. The warm suction of her body enveloping his length, her hips moving in slow, sultry circles as she stirs her brew with his cock.

He feels his orgasm rising and shudders, like she does, when he slaps her ass and lifts his hips, gyrating his pubis into her clit, making her come again and again and again.

He wipes his release from his abdomen with his discarded T-shirt and tucks her story into his pillow. He wraps his arms around it, imagining it is her and falls asleep knowing that a thousand words is worth more than any picture.

*   *   *

She lies awake in bed, her naked flesh glowing in the light of the full moon. After being jolted from her fantasy by the horny grouse that morning, she ended up spending much of the afternoon peering through binoculars at a mating pair of red tail hawks nesting around their cabin. She hates that her mate has to leave her just as spring is bursting from the bud and every living thing on the planet is having sex. Except for her.

She closes her eyes and goes back to his beach knowing he is probably sleeping by now. She lays her head on his thigh and takes him into her mouth. She lets him fill her throat, deeper than she can actually take him, before pumping it like the male grouse. She swallows, encouraging her throat to squeeze all around him as one hand jacks his shaft and the other lightly tickles his testicles. When she feels his body tightening, his orgasm rising, she doesn't stop and keeps sucking until she feels him come. In her fantasy, she never gags, and swallows his load effortlessly as her throat continues to convulse around him.

Her hands drift over her moonlit skin, down to her bush that she hasn't shaved since he left her three weeks ago. The hair holds the musky scent of her lust that drifts across her belly taunting her nose with its need. She explores her folds gently at first but then with increasing vigor until she is slapping herself. It surprises her, the pussy-spanking, as he calls it. He's the one with the sadistic streak that loves the sound of flesh smacking on flesh. He's the one who taught her how ecstatic a little pain nudged up to pleasure can feel. She rolls over, buries her face into his pillow and impales herself on her peace-sign fingers, circling her hips, grinding her clit into her palm wishing it was the hard surface of his abdominals. When she reaches back and slaps her ass, it's not the same, but she feels a small shudder of release.

She rolls onto her back, letting the moonlight caress her belly as her palm floats across her breasts. She wonders if he ever feels her coming to his beach, or if he has received her story yet. As if in response, her fingers hone in on her nipple and lightly pinch.

She smiles and rolls to her side. His arms, reaching from California, wrap around her, pulling her close.

They fall asleep remembering.

CHAPTER FOURTEEN

June 2007
Bare

I'M BEING SEDUCED.

Her voice, light as a downy feather, floats across the meadow, tickling the morning fog of my consciousness.

Come.

I let myself be lured from a second cup of tea and end up standing in front of the sliding glass door of the cabin, staring out at her. She is bare, wrapped in nothing but a cloudy white shawl to ward off the chill that still clings to the mountains, despite tomorrow's summer solstice. I am wrapped in nothing but my adventurer's large hooded sweatshirt that engulfs me in his absence. As I slide the door open, I feel the morning rise up my legs, making my nipples stiffen against his hoodie's soft cotton lining.

Sit.

She directs my gaze to the weathered deck at my feet as if she is patting the seat of a sofa beside her. I reach for a blanket and the rolled-up sleeping pad that doubles as my meditation cushion, and position them over the splintery wood. I pull my hood over my head and sit, monk-like, before her, the front edge of the blanket tucked over my crossed legs for warmth.

Breathe.

I draw the coolness of the dawn through my nostrils, into my belly, and feel it rise up my torso like the mist that now hovers near her peak. The crown of my head lifts toward the sky and I mimic the aspens across the meadow as I straighten and elongate my spine. I exhale and my face softens. My shoulders drop away from my ears.

In the winter, this mountain seduces my man, enticing him to mount her and ski her powdery avalanche chutes. But her fluffy winter coat has melted into whitewater, taking him and his passion for kayaking with it. In his absence, she amuses herself with me.

I take in her unassuming beauty, a simple, treed triangular peak. The bald spot near her summit is divided by a diagonal line of pines, making it look like an oval-shaped yin and yang symbol, reminding me that there is balance in the opposites. Right now I am alone, the yin of Mount Hailey's bare peak seducing me back to my meditation cushion, my yoga mat, myself. All winter I shared this 800-square-foot cabin with my backcountry skier, fully engaged in the yang of climbing her snowy summit. I think of us, after a day of skiing, sipping red wine and stretching in front of the woodstove, our wool base layers sliding from our bodies until we are naked and entwined. Longing threatens to sweep over me like an avalanche.

Stay.

Her voice is softer than a whisper, barely distinguishable from my own. I reel my thoughts in, to my breath, to the sun that is creeping across the meadow to my perch on the deck. I bring my attention to the liquid silver clinging to blades of wild grass, remnants of last night's thunderstorm. The meadow is freshly showered and littered with a confetti of wildflowers. The wood of the deck is dark, saturated, a rare thing in June in the high country desert. But the humidity feels heavy across my shoulders and my spine feels too tired to hold them up. I don't want to sit here. I want another cup of tea. I want to feel the heat of his body wrapped around me. I want…

Gratitude.

She nudges and I notice the whining, grasping nature of my thoughts. Gratitude, I know, soothes like a balm, and is the perfect place to start a reluctant contemplative practice. As I inhale, I remember to be thankful for the air that moves in and out of my lungs; for the health and vitality of my body even though right now I feel so tired and stiff I can't imagine sitting still like this for another twenty minutes. I give thanks for the deep connection I share with my husband, even though we are a thousand miles apart. The contractive feeling of longing for him shifts and my chest grows warm and expansive. The words 'thank you' form audibly on my lips. If you were to ask me who the 'you' is that I am thanking, I would have to say that this mountain in front of me, on the verge of summer, adorned now with the orange sherbet-colored clouds of a sunrise sums it up the best.

I notice movement: a bluebird flying across the meadow, a chipmunk scurrying through the sage. My stomach rumbles. I mentally gather ingredients for a spinach and feta omelet, wondering if I have any fresh tomatoes. I begin to make a list of supplies I will need when I go into town for groceries.

Come back.

I catch myself, not present, drifting away from the morning unfolding between me and my favorite mountain. The clouds around her peak are reaching out to me now like long, rosy fingers. I am amazed that I can be sitting here witnessing a scene worthy of an artist's canvas and my thoughts drift to the grocery store. Daydreaming about a mountain sunrise to escape waiting in line at the grocery store makes sense. But not the opposite. Here's a mouthful: being mindful of not being mindful is the definition of being mindful.

Close your eyes.

As I do, I feel my sacrum melt towards the earth. My shoulders follow. I exhale into a deep, quiet calm.

This is what matters. I sit, effortlessly, basking in that truth for what could be minutes or an hour, I don't know or care. I sit until my cross-legged position gets uncomfortable and my feet go numb.

Stretch.

I slide the blanket off my legs and extend them, rolling my ankles around as I push the hood of my sweatshirt back. Sunlight dapples the deck now, warming me as I roll my head slowly from side to side and circle my arms overhead. As I flow into a simple seated twist, I see my reflection, compact and blonde, in the sliding glass door behind me. Mount Hailey's image floats right above my shoulder, a perfect representation of witness consciousness, a concept I first experienced at my yoga teacher training at Kripalu and one that Eckhart Tolle reminded me of again the other day as I re-read *A New Earth*.

For me, the witness feels like a smaller, wiser version of myself that perches on my shoulder, a meditative mini-me that identifies my unconscious habits before I launch into them. I hear, *Hmmm, I feel defensive* instead of launching into a tirade of self-righteousness.

In the early years of my love affair with my adventurer, in that intoxicating, infatuation phase that lasted about three years for us, I found that being out here at the cabin when he was gone courting whitewater was almost unbearable. Our love nest felt so empty. The Pathetic Wife, weighted down with all her emotional baggage packed with rejection and abandonment issues, moped. My Yoga Teacher came to the rescue, determined to make the most of the forced retreat, with a regimen of yoga, meditation and readings on Buddhist philosophy. When my witness showed up and gave some much-needed perspective on the situation, I ended up at my keyboard to sort it all out. I began to write these stories. In time, I rediscovered the joy of being alone. But actually, I wasn't alone at all. I wasn't, after all, the only one who'd been abandoned.

Breathe.

I inhale, filling my twist with breath and then releasing it with an exhalation. I lean forward and relax into a forward bend inviting my breath now into the tight muscles of my lower back, willing them to soften, warming my bare thighs with an exhalation. As my torso rises, I move into a twist on the other side, and face her directly

At times, Mount Hailey is like the perfect girlfriend, sitting with me in silence, holding space for my wild torrent of thoughts, not judging, not interrupting, not talking. Other times, she is like Mount Olympus, housing the gods of creativity who lounge around her peak and shoot inspiration at me like fiery arrows.

Flow.

I release my twist and move on to my hands and knees, circling my hips around before I push back into child's pose. As I bow forward and surrender, I understand that it isn't just this mountain in front of me that inspires, but the whole of what she represents, which is so huge I'm not sure I can even define it. I slither into cobra pose and invite the breath up to my heart and throat before I lift my core back and flow into downward dog.

Sit.

I drop my knees and sit in diamond poise, grounding my tailbone, my thoughts. As I do, a realization dawns on me like the sun. I fell in love so hard I got the breath knocked out of me, so it is no wonder I lost my connection to consciously acknowledging its presence. I was too busy gasping in ecstatic wonder.

Initially, we wanted to share everything. But I am learning that even in the most passionate, soulful relationship, there are places you can't, and shouldn't go together. I don't follow him to Class V whitewater. He doesn't share my meditation cushion. We have different bridges that lead to the same place. Exploring our individual passions allows us to tap in deeply, so when we come back together, the marriage of our energies allow us to transcend even higher.

Inhale.

As I draw in the sunlight-infused air, it feels like it is infiltrating my brain, enlightening my thoughts.

In my attempts to figure out this *ménage a trois* dynamic of my marriage, I've personified my man's passion as a femme fatale 'other'. But he was married to adventure long before I came along. Perhaps I am the third, the one that has been added and seduced into the fold.

But I've been entranced by mountains all my life. As a child, I remember picking out a folder for my schoolwork that had a picture of a mountain stream on it. My favorite doodle was a jagged line of mountains with a sun rising out from it. When I was eighteen, I left my family home in the Midwest and headed to Colorado for college. I knew, in a way my eighteen-year-old self couldn't articulate, that I needed to live closer to wildness. Her seduction intensified and after my sophomore year I dropped out of college because all I really wanted to study was her and the euphoria of melding into a mountain on skis.

She holds me, scolds me, spanks and soothes. She's the diamond glint of sun on snow and the threat of an avalanche just below the surface. This morning, she is my soft-spoken witness, stripped down for summer.

I pull off my man's hoodie and sit, bare, before her.

There has to be a word that encapsulates all of this...essence, eden, soul, spirit, chi, gaia, goddess, God, guru...but nothing quite does.

I lie back and move into fish pose, lifting my sternum, my throat to the sky. My head slides until I am resting on my crown, draining it of thought.

And then the word I am searching for brushes across my lips like a soft kiss.

Muse.

CHAPTER FIFTEEN

July 2007
Dear River

DEAR RIVER,

I thought we had an agreement: *We'll share. We'll share. We'll share.*
I'm doing my part. I've been working hard to keep The Pathetic
Wife at bay, graciously handing over our kayaker in May, knowing I
won't see his ruggedly handsome face back home until mid-July.
I've learned to let him have his fun while you are frothing and wet
since you eventually dry up and go away.

But now you want more.

I see what you are doing. You are captivating his scientific mind
with your ecological issues: the diminished salmon and elk
populations on the California Salmon River; the possibility of
removing the dams on the neighboring Klamath River. During my
two-week visit to Northern California this year, he was distracted
with thoughts of you. His mind churned behind his sunglasses,
trying to figure out how he could get grants for research or maybe
even funding for a Ph.D., which means at least four years,
researching, studying, writing about *you*. Just when I thought his
passion for you might mellow as he progressed in his scientific
career, you sucked him in even deeper, trying to transform his
seasonal kayak obsession into a year-round professional pursuit.

You clever bitch.

I must say, I'm quite impressed. My tactics to keep here him in
Colorado didn't pan out. I rooted for the Ph.D. program to study

wolves and elk in Yellowstone with course work at the university an hour from here. Just one hour! But fair enough, that was a little greedy because there isn't that much river activity around here, only a short window to run the North Platte and the Encampment rivers in the spring.

So I really don't blame you for trying.

But you're making me nervous. He's been meeting with members of the Karuk Indian tribe, who are lobbying for the removal of the dams on the Klamath; rowing rafts for the annual meeting of the local watershed council; getting invited to parties with the staff of the Salmon River Restoration Council. After he dropped me at the airport he went to the assessor's office to research property for sale on the Salmon River.

How are you finagling all this?

I sit here alone at our cabin wondering what is going to happen with our lives and feel oddly threatened that it is you, not us, who is navigating our course.

But let's get a few things straight, River. We are a package deal, he and I. We've been given one of the rarest of gifts: a blissful, sexy marriage. Sure, he gets off on your Class V rapids in a way I'll never understand, but the tongue of your rapid can't dance with his in a passionate French kiss. Your tongue, thank God, can't suck cock.

Obviously, he'd be miserable without either one of us, so we might as well give up this tug of war. Besides, his heart is huge; there is plenty of passion for both of us.

The Science Seductress has upset the balance. Grad school stole time away from both of us. I realize he shows up at your shores with his laptop and drafts of his thesis due. I know you had to give him up early last year when he rushed home to protest the leasing of our mineral rights for oil and gas development. Believe me, I understand your hunger for more. I was relegated to weekend conjugal visits these past two years of grad school. His nose was buried in wildlife statistics a lot more than my bush.

We are both feeling needy and greedy for more. Since we are in the same boat, we might as well paddle together.

I'm trying to open myself to you, I really am. You, with your achingly beautiful green water, bordered by puffy, pinked-lipped snapdragons. You, with your wild tangle of blackberry bush and turquoise swimming holes.

But living by you means leaving here. These mountains have been my home for thirteen years. Our homestead has become my sanctuary, surrounded by trusted friends. Mount Hailey meditates with me every morning. Ute Ridge has vignettes of our love affair penciled on her summit register. And the vista in between, where we got married, is nothing less than a portal. Every time I go up there, I add a rock to the cairn where we had our wedding ceremony. I send out gratitude and intentions to the surrounding peaks. I know that I am heard.

I feel so connected, so free under this endless blue sky. But admittedly, the forecast here could be bleak. The oil and gas company that bought the mineral lease to our land has the right to drill here. The pine beetle epidemic is turning our evergreen forests to rust. It is currently creeping like an angry rash up the east side of Mount Hailey, killing the trees that hold the powder stashes that we ski all winter. A single strike of lightning could turn it all to flame, smoke and ash.

It could all be too unbearable to watch.

So maybe it is time to fly from this cozy nest. I realize that as we move into the fourth year of our marriage, our love is shifting away from the energy of the sky with its fiery sunsets and falling stars and moving downward, grounding towards the earth where it can take root and continue to grow. We are both cultivating new careers and trying to create a vision for mid-life.

The lower altitude of California would definitely be better for aging. We could grow our own organic food and add wild salmon to our freezer of elk. New adventures await, exploring your currents and the nearby coast. So why do I hesitate?

Well, you *are* a bit intimidating. For starters, I still feel like a nervous guppy even after two stints at kayak school. And there is that incredible pull you have on my husband, and you've been tugging hard lately. I know you need a brilliant scientific mind like his to unravel what is happening to your salmon and elk populations. He is captivated by the challenge. I want to support him, but I have to figure out a way of doing it without losing myself.

I look down at my wedding ring: a white gold band with carved mountains, inlaid with two slivers of Salmon River jade. As I spin it around my finger, I think of the ceremony we wrote, based on the theme of mountains and rivers. Suddenly, I am digging through my files for a copy. As I read it, words jump off the page, slapping me in the face:

... open to the unexpected in life and navigate change gracefully...

... our marriage, a passionate dance amidst our present and future homes in the mountains and rivers of Colorado and Northern California...

... fully-funded grad school project in wildlife and river ecology...getting erotica published...

I shake my head, stunned. How could I have forgotten all this in just four years?

You're not the clever bitch. I am the oblivious one.

My hand goes to my throat and caresses the smooth green stone that I wear, a smaller version of the river talisman that hangs from my husband's neck. I adorn myself with stones from your river bed. I stood at a portal on my wedding day and put out this intention. And then I start accusing you when it starts to manifest?

There is no tug of war going on here. I am the only one holding the rope, tethering myself to the familiar. But why? The familiar isn't really working anymore. I sit at our cabin in the middle of July missing my husband. My eyes are red and watery. My ears itch from allergies. My neck is sore from giving too many deep-tissue massages. I married a man with a huge sense of adventure, but what has happened to my own?

Have I become too much like these mountains around me, stationary and still? But as I continue to spin my wedding ring around my finger, I realize that our vision, like its design, is for mountains *and* rivers. It's not an either or thing. I really don't have to give up anything.

I'm just adding more of you.

You embody everything I'm trying to convey in my stories: passion, flow, beauty, adventure. I know you are complicated, believe me, and understanding you takes more than a week in my boat every year. Certainly, living at your shore would give me the opportunity to become more intimate with you. We aren't so different. My body is a river of blood, lymph and emotion. I have my boiling eddy lines and turbulent holes too.

Perhaps you could help me cultivate this dream of sharing my words. I could focus on writing there, since I don't know what other kind of work I would do. When doubt creeps in and the words get stuck, I could slip into your current, tap into your flow.

If I were there, I would convey this to you personally, float my naked body in one of your swimming holes and trust. But I'm not, so I am sending this letter to my husband and ask that he perform this ritual.

I imagine him releasing this small bundle of new moon sage from our cabin into your current when he says goodbye to you in August. I've wrapped strands of my blond hair around it and want him to add a few strands of his own so all four elements of our vision are present and integrated: mountains, rivers, husband, wife. I've included a bluebird feather to represent the courage to fly.

As we move into our fourth year of marriage, we will share, all four of us, even deeper. You will always be his mistress but perhaps instead of being my nemesis, you could become my muse. But there I go, missing the obvious again.

You already are.

CHAPTER SIXTEEN

October 2007
Kneeling to Prey

THE ROUGHNESS OF MY hunter's two-day beard grazes my cheek as his lips brush up against mine. I smell coffee on his exhalation and feel the weight of his hand as it slowly contours the hills and valley of my ribcage, waist and hips beneath our Hudson Bay wool blanket. His touch gathers speed down the runway of my leg, takes flight at my ankle and then he is gone, blending into the pre-dawn darkness.

The next time I stir, I awaken to the sound of a bull elk bugling, a haunting, primal call that challenges other bulls to a duel. They snort, piss and crash their antlers together, competing for a herd of cow elk in estrous.

It's a sexy time of year to be an elk.

It's also a very dangerous time. My man is one of hundreds who woke before dawn for the opening day of hunting season. I lie in the loft of our cabin watching the day break in a blaze of pink and even though our freezer is low on elk steaks, I can't help but root for the animals.

I slide out of bed and into a satin robe and head down stairs to make a cup of tea. I find the leopard-print lace thong that made its debut last night, draped over my hunter's empty coffee cup. Its pink lace bisected my ass for all of thirty seconds before he pounced, grabbed them in his teeth and slid them down slowly, making the legs of my 5'2" frame feel as long as a supermodel's. I smile as I step back into them, knowing it was eighteen dollars well spent.

The fall morning is heating up under the Colorado sun, making it much too hot for the hunting to be very good. I lounge on the deck with my tea, untie my sash and let my robe fall open. I feel every inch the sex kitten as I stroke my leopard spots, knowing my hunter will be home very soon.

An hour later when he still isn't home, I can't quit thinking of the recent report of a mountain lion attack. A local bow hunter, positioning himself to take a shot on a bull elk, felt the hairs on his neck rise and turned to find a mountain lion stalking him. He raised his arms, yelled, and did everything you are supposed to do to discourage a cat, but to no avail. He drew his bow and shot the 150-pound male in the chest as it sprang toward him. There is poetic justice there, the hunter becoming prey, but not when my hunter is late for breakfast.

When I see movement across the meadow in the gold-coined aspen leaves, I purr with relief as my hunter steps out with a front quarter of an elk slung over his shoulder.

I watch him hike up the knoll to our cabin and am reminded of a red wine-filled night in Queenstown, New Zealand, when a sassy British woman in our group directed the conversation towards sexy professions and asked everyone at the table what they did for a living. My husband won the last glass of Pinot Noir with his trio of entries: hunting guide, raft guide and whitewater kayak instructor.

I must admit he looks sexy as hell with his pecs and biceps bulging beneath his camouflage shirt as he drops a slab of wild game at my feet. I half-expect him to grab me by the hair and pull me back to bed, but when our eyes meet, there is no passion there. Just death. His brown eyes look as flat as the dried blood on his hands.

"I'm going to take the truck and pick up the rest," he says as he pulls a skinning blade from his pocket and slaps it in my hand. He turns and leaves without even a glance at my leopard spots.

I watch his back and wonder what happened to the man I fell asleep with last night, the tender lover with the velvet tongue who drenched my nipples and clitoris with Grand Marnier and licked until I came. As he opens the door to his truck, I find myself staring at his hands that from now until Thanksgiving will be raw and scabbed from carving up elk carcasses. How could they be the same hands that caress the silky flesh between my thighs with such gentleness and finesse?

I marvel at the dichotomy: my lover, my killer. As his truck disappears into the trees, I realize that it's testosterone that drives them both. The same biochemical that drove him to tear my leopard spots off last night has him not even noticing them today. I hear a gunshot echo off to the west and realize the mountain air is literally pulsing with testosterone right now. The moose, elk and antelope are all in rut. Hundreds of armed men are in the woods trying to kill them. I look down across satin and lace at the hunk of bloody elk carcass lying at my feet.

I really need to shift gears.

I strip and change into a pair of old jeans, a T-shirt and a John Deere baseball cap that I pull low over a messy ponytail. Back on the deck, I do a few yoga breaths and visualize all the testosterone-infused air moving deeply into my lungs. I catch my reflection in the sliding glass door and cup my hand around my crotch, adjusting my labial lips inside my thong like a couple of testicles.

I flick open the skinning knife, grab a piece of hide and start cutting.

By late afternoon, the elk is skinned and hung in the shed to cure. We've butchered the finest cuts of meat, the back straps and tenderloins, into steaks. My hunter grabs a beer and pours a glass of Merlot for me.

"I'm beat." He pulls off his camo shirt and pants and leaves them in a blood-spattered heap on the floor. He slides into our wooden rocker that is draped with an antelope hide to cover its desperate need for refinishing. "I need a shower," he says as he takes another pull from his beer and closes his eyes.

I'm suddenly aware that I smell like a dead elk, so I add my jeans and T-shirt to the pile. My man is too tired to notice or care that I am sitting on the couch across from him in nothing but my leopard thong. I sip my Merlot and watch my man in this rare inert state. Like the young bull elk we've been handling all day, there is no excess on my hunter's frame. His body is dark, lean and linear. I, on the other hand, am a study of pale curves. My palm traces the arch of my hip and slides down across my spots. Even though I've scrubbed my hands with bleach water, dried elk blood clings to the cuticles. I flex my fingers, testing their strength and feel an overwhelming desire to scrape them down the pelt of dark hair that cascades down my husband's abdomen. He is tired and matted with elk blood. Such easy prey.

I drain my glass of Merlot that is warm and heavy, like blood, on my tongue. It further incites my primal thirst. I slither off the couch and move slowly on all fours across the room. When a low moan rumbles in the back of my throat, my hunter opens one eye and catches me mid-stalk, licking my lips and eyeing his crotch.

He doesn't want this.

I do.

I tug one wool sock and then the other from his feet and drag my bloody claws down his legs with his silk boxer briefs. I push his legs apart and sink my teeth into the striated belly of his quadriceps.

"Owww! Hey, what's gotten into you?"

My gaze focuses on his groin and the sac tucked humbly behind his relaxed cock. It looks so unassuming back there, but I know better.

My hunter watches me as I watch him. Despite his fatigue, his cock thickens from my penetrating gaze, rising slowly, magnificently, but it is the fleshy pouch hiding behind the scene that is really capturing my attention. His cache of maleness draws me like a calico to catnip.

"This..." I say as I cup his sac in my hands, reverently, like a chalice, "...has gotten into me." The moon is hanging half-full in the sky and like me, is midway through its monthly cycle. My own testosterone level, however slight, is at its monthly peak. Factor in that I've been breathing rut-ridden air all day while my hands were immersed in the blood of a bull elk. My testosterone level is at an all-time high.

I shove his cock out of the way, bury my face into the crease of his upper thigh and inhale. Musk. Blood. Sweat. My nose circles all around his scrotum vacuuming up his scent. My elbows wrap around his knees and slide him and the antelope hide to the edge of the chair until his testicles hang free. I crouch down and toy with them, humming and purring as I rub my cheeks, lips and chin against his source, greedy for more of his male essence.

I run my tongue over my dry lips and porous teeth that I know are stained red from the Merlot. My jaw opens wide and I begin to devour him, sucking one testis and then the other into my mouth like gum balls. I roll them around my mouth until they are slick, and let my tongue drift up and down his shaft until it glistens. As one hand caresses and tickles his balls, the other begins to squeeze and jack.

I rock the chair with my shoulder, letting its momentum move my hand up and down his cock. My predatory gaze creeps across the hard plateau of his belly and up to his heavy-lidded brown eyes.

I bare my wine-stained teeth and purposefully graze them over the head of his cock as it slides in and out of my mouth. I take him deep into my throat and swallow. Twice. I slide him out, letting my teeth graze his length, and wait for his eyes to meet mine again. When they do, I open my mouth wide and slap his rod against my tongue.

I bring a finger to my mouth, slather it in saliva and slide my hand beneath him until I find his opening. The urge to penetrate, to fuck, to thrust, burns at my clit.

He gasps as I push up against his sphincter. He is tight, tender here, and I force myself to back off, realizing this is how it must be for him when he wakes up rock-hard-horny and I am sleepy, shy and dry. I try to recall how he caresses me into arousal and try to duplicate his gentleness and finesse, listening, as he does, to the signals of body language and breath. There's a bottle of lube in the loft but I know if I make a move towards it, this moment will be lost. I improvise with more saliva and feel his glutes relax into my hand. I lightly circle and stroke his opening, despite my nearly overwhelming urge to thrust in. I take the honey quality of his moan for confirmation that I've got the pressure right and I channel my aggression toward his cock, continuing to work him with teeth, tongue and palm.

I feel his balls tighten and encourage him to plunge even deeper into my throat that, thanks to the wine, is even more relaxed and accommodating to his length. As I feel his orgasm rising, I can no longer deny myself. My finger pushes in. He gasps in surprise, pain, pleasure—I'm not sure. When his sphincter relaxes its grip, I thrust and suck in a coordinated rhythm until he bucks his hips and explodes, hot and slippery, into my mouth.

I pull back, thinking that if I swallow I just may have chest hair by morning. I gather his cum on my tongue and let it spill over my lips and chin. But then I have a flash of the four flanks of meat hanging outside. We have another full day of butchering ahead.

I lie back and rub his testo-juice into my breastbone, letting it all soak in.

CHAPTER SEVENTEEN

April/May 2008
A Royal Spanking

I'M GETTING SPANKED. By a queen.

Oh, how I wish she was a gorgeous drag queen, laughing in her husky voice as she punishes me for sneaking into her blue glitter mascara. Or better yet, Cate Blanchett dressed in full queen regalia slapping my reddening buttocks with her delicate white-skinned hand. But right now, I'd gladly offer up my bare bum to stern old Elizabeth armed with a royal wooden paddle.

Anything, really, but this.

Because I disrespected a wild and unpredictable queen, the queen of all river trips, the 297-mile stretch of the Colorado River that runs through the Grand Canyon. And when this queen decided to teach me a lesson, she started spanking so hard she's taking my breath away. As my body tumbles and churns beneath the aqua-colored water of one of her more formidable rapids, I am starting to wonder if she's ever going to give it back.

I made the mistake of using the Q-word in reference to myself, repeatedly, right in front of her. But I really did feel like royalty, perched on the back of an eighteen-foot raft, barely getting wet as my man navigated us through the rapids of the Grand Canyon's Inner Gorge. As if anticipating our arrival, the canyon wildflowers were in full bloom, draped like garland along the shoreline. I even had a ten-foot high, red-and-gold dragon flag rigged to the bow and a throne of sorts in the stern: my husband's upside down kayak braced by our dry bags and sleeping pads.

"Only the most skilled river knight gets to row the queen down the river," I joked as he stood up in the boat to get a read on the upcoming rapid.

"Well, we can't have the queen getting wet." He spun the boat and made a backward approach into the foamy, white water.

"She is already soaking wet between her regal thighs because her river knight is so incredibly hot." He pushed hard with his left oar, positioning our bow forward and perpendicular to a crashing wave. Besides the inside fabric of my bikini bottom, the only part of me that was damp at the bottom of that rapid was the underarms of my polypro shirt, a combination of nervous excitement and the heat of the late-April desert sun.

I had no idea at the time that the *real* queen in this scenario was getting a little tired of my impropriety. And the luck that landed us this last-minute, highly-coveted Grand Canyon permit was starting to run out.

* * *

My husband called me from New Mexico where he was presenting his master's thesis at a wildlife biology conference. Unlike the last time we talked, when the beige walls of his hotel room were closing in on him, he sounded happy and upbeat. After twenty years of being an outdoor adventure guide, his transition into the scientific arena had its challenges primarily because he had a hard time sitting still and being indoors, two things he'd been doing all week.

"What are ya doin'?" he asked.

"I've got one client walking out the door and another one pulling up." In other words, I had no time to talk.

He couldn't contain himself and blurted out his news anyway. "I just won the lottery for a Grand Canyon permit."

"No way," I leaned my hip against the corner of my desk. It took him ten years on a waiting list to get a permit for his last Grand Canyon trip, an event that took place before I met him.

"It's a last-minute cancellation permit. We launch April 20th."

There was a pause as I searched for my calendar, trying to figure out what day it was.

"That's ten days from now," he explained.

"Holy shit."

He laughed. "It's crazy isn't it? Do you think we can do it?"

In the circles we run, ski and paddle in, there's a creed: If you get a chance to go on the Grand Canyon, you drop everything and go.

"We have to," I said.

"I know," he said excitedly.

"Are we going to invite anyone else?"

"I don't think we have time."

The idea of just the two of us on a raft exploring one of the Seven Natural Wonders of the World sounded incredibly romantic, a once-in-a-lifetime kind of adventure. But the Grand Canyon has some of the heaviest whitewater in North America. Unlike my husband who's been running rivers for half his adult life, I can read Greek better than I can read a river.

"Can we do it alone?" I asked, hating the Nervous Nellie tone in my voice.

"I rowed the entire thing in 2001," he said confidently. "It's big water, Class III. No problem." (For those of you who ski, Class III whitewater is like a blue run at a ski area.)

And then he sealed the deal. "Besides, who else could possibly be more fun than just the two of us?"

My Hopeless Romantic melted right into the chair because I could think of at least thirty friends that would be a blast to take down the river. She shoved the Nervous Nellie out the door as my next client entered, with the assurance that our adventurer lives to run Class V white water, the equivalent of a double black diamond ski run. The Grand Canyon would be like a water park for him.

But what I've since realized is when highly-skilled adventurer athletes are injured or killed, it isn't usually on the hard stuff. Accidents often happen on the easier stuff, when their guard is down.

And my knight's guard was down on day ten of the trip.

Although, it might be more accurate to say that the river seduced his armor from him, one piece at time, the day before when we ran the first part of the Inner Gorge with the Maynards, a sixteen-person trip from Maine. One of the oarsmen, Kirk, described them as an AARP trip, since most of their group was in their fifties and sixties. We shared a launch date, a campsite and one of their gourmet dinners. We'd become fast friends.

Our two trips converged again on day nine on the shores of Hance Rapid, the first of the formidable Inner Gorge rapids. A few of the Maynard boatmen were Grand Canyon rookies, so they were playing it safe, taking the easiest line and skirting the rapid all together to avoid the most turbulent whitewater.

"I didn't come to the Grand Canyon to miss all the rapids," my guide said as we jumped in our raft and took the harder line through the guts of the rapid, purposefully hitting the big waves and going for the ultimate thrill.

The Maynards cheered us on, and suddenly in our forties, we were the young bucks, the adventurous couple much like Glen and Bessie Hyde who ran the canyon on their honeymoon in 1928. Never mind that those two disappeared without a trace after the rapid at mile 232 and were never seen again. Halfway through the gorge, our egos were as inflated as our rubber raft.

While scouting Hermit, the second to the last rapid of the gorge, we decided to stop and make camp.

"Are you sure you don't want to continue on and run Crystal rapid with us?" Kirk asked. "It's a great warm day for running big water." There was a subtle note of concern in his voice, something neither of us picked up on because we were so busy unstrapping my husband's kayak from our raft, so he could play in a big surf wave at the bottom of the rapid.

Within minutes, my knight mounted his steed and charged through Hermit, so he could provide safety for the Maynards as they came through. Having lost my throne, I became a lady-in-waiting and stood on shore and cheered for everyone as they navigated the rapid. My knight paddled up through the eddies and re-ran the lower part of the rapid, again and again, gracefully leaning and turning, waltzing with his queen and her five-foot high waves.

The next morning was cloudy and cool as we stood on the rocks scouting Crystal, a rapid that was ranked a nine in our guidebook. Just to confuse novices like me, there is a 1-10 rating scale used for the Grand Canyon rapids instead of the standard I-V categorization. Regardless, that put Crystal right up there in the black diamond category, so we pulled over above the rapid to take a look.

It was big, the largest rapid we'd seen yet, with a big churning hydraulic hole at the top that made my stomach rise up to my throat. The roar of the whitewater was so loud I could hardly hear my guide as he pointed out a line through the right side of the rapid that avoided the hole and skirted most of the crashing waves. It was the safest route, the route the Maynards undoubtedly took.

But then the glassy smooth water pouring into the top of the rapid, the tongue as it is called, reached to the shore and licked up one of my husband's testicles and down the other. In a sultry whisper that only the most experienced boatmen can hear, the queen summoned her knight.

"Hey, big boy," she purred as she tossed her wild white mane against the canyon walls on the left side of the river, sending up a frothy splash of whitewater that affected my husband much like cleavage spilling out from a tight corset. "Come on over here. Not many do. Only real men like you."

She stirred up in him a potent cocktail of pheromones— testosterone, adrenaline, endorphins — and served up my ideal of a sexy man: fearless, strong, and impassioned by the power of a river.

We were mesmerized: him by her and me by the effect she was having on him. Suddenly, we were engaged in a high-stakes threesome and the river was the only one who knew it.

Under her spell, we jumped into our raft. I climbed onto my throne in the back, somehow believing since he was worthy of her left line, that somehow through association I was too. I think she took enormous pleasure in showing me just how wrong I was as our raft got sideways against the canyon wall. She reached up and in an instant I was dethroned. She pulled me deep into her tight cold embrace and started spanking.

When I finally emerged, I heard my name. I turned and saw my guide on top of our upside-down raft five feet upstream from where I was gasping for air.

"Swim," he said in a tone of voice that frightened me even more. At home, I swim a mile, three to four days a week, so I broke into a powerful, freestyle stroke. But my one-hundred-and-fifteen pounds soaking wet was still so much lighter than our raft. The current kept pulling me farther away.

"Come on, you can do it," he said and what I heard was: you have to do it. I tried again, and again, but made no progress. He couldn't help me since any rope he could throw or oar he could extend were all strapped to the underneath side of the boat.

"I'm not getting anywhere," I said between breaths. The forty-five degree water was sapping my strength. "I can't." I hated the sound of those words coming from my mouth.

I looked downstream and saw the horizon line and realized there was more whitewater coming.

"Grab my foot." I turned back to the sound of my guide's voice. He was in the water, holding onto the boat with one hand while stretching the length of his six-foot frame out to me. I summoned the strength, took a few more strokes and barely got a grip on the rubber sole of his Chaco sandal. He bent his knee, grabbed my lifejacket and put my hand on one of the raft's side handles.

"Hold on," he said as we moved through a wave train. I was expecting to go under again, so I took a deep breath, but mercifully it didn't happen. He hoisted himself up onto the bottom of the raft and pulled me up after him. My whole body was shaking—from fear, adrenaline, exhaustion, and cold.

"They're coming." He grabbed my hand.

I followed his gaze upstream and saw the Maynards' yellow rafts deploying from their camp below Crystal. The 'old guys' were coming to our rescue.

They reached us and towed us to shore before we hit the next rapid and it took all eighteen of us to flip over our raft. Everyone cheered when our flag rose up and caught in the wind.

The women hugged me: I'd just survived their greatest fear. Tom, one of the two lobstermen in the group, handed me a fleece jacket that came down to my knees. Scott, the most seasoned boatmen on the trip, asked my husband what happened.

"We went left..." he began and I saw Scott cringe. Sue, the woman who was currently hugging me said, "Don't feel bad. Our guidebook said that even the most experienced guides flip there. It's that eddy fence by the wall." I'd never heard the term 'eddy fence' before, but I knew it was what held me under and spanked.

My husband and I shivered despite the warmth and kindness of these wonderful people. I looked at him and when our eyes met, the realization was harsh. We took the hard line through one of the canyon's biggest rapids, by ourselves, with no support. We climbed on our raft and our bamboo flagpole that once stood so tall and proud was broken near the top, making our flag flop crookedly to one side, like a jester's hat, an appropriate banner for a couple of fools.

Later, we were sitting in camp, licking our wounds and applying the balm of beer. After three hours of sorting through soggy gear, we finally managed to hang it all up to dry. In an attempt to regain our dignity, we repaired the flag. I stitched up the holes with our mini sewing kit while my husband duct-taped tamarisk branch supports to the flagpole. The cheap Mexican beer had the desired effect and we had both gotten buzzed enough that we could talk about flipping our raft like it was a fun thing to do.

Flipping isn't that big of a deal for my guide. When he takes clients down Gore Canyon, the Class IV-V stretch of this same river near our home in Colorado, it's just part of a day's work. He's good at it, sees it coming, and like today often lands on the bottom of the raft dry as a bone. But as my husband, he feels terrible that he got me in over my head. I'm trying to play it cool and not let it leak out that I share the sentiment.

"I was starting to get worried when I didn't see you come up," he admits. "I was afraid you were trapped under the raft. How long do you think you were under?"

"Like how many hours?" My attempt at humor lands flat on his face. "I guess you mean seconds then. Let me think..." I hold up my thumb and begin to count. "One: I'm in the water." I extend my index finger "Two: The water is aqua-colored. That's good. I'm no longer under the boat. Three: I should be popping up any time now. Four: *I really need a breath*. Five..." I extend my pinkie finger and we both notice that my hand is quivering. I swallow and try to keep it from traveling up to my voice. "Five: I feel water seeping between my lips, so I clamp them shut tighter."

I need my other hand, so I set my beer in the sand and extend my thumb. "Six: I'm really churning. I must be stuck in the eddy line. Seven: Shit. Eight: Stay calm, stay calm. Nine: Please..." I am running out of fingers and both my hands tremble as I hold them open, facing him. I think there were a few more panicked pleas in there, but I don't feel like revisiting it anymore, and my guide has suffered enough. "Ten: I hear you call my name and yell, 'Swim' in a tone of voice that scares the shit out of me. So, ten seconds, I guess." I try to sound matter-of-fact, but I can't help it, a tear leaks out. The rapid sucked the sunglasses off my face, so I am wearing his back-up pair. They are big for my face and dark. They say the eyes are the windows to the soul. Right now, I am grateful for the shades.

He kneels in the sand in front of me and presses his palms against mine. "I'm sorry," he says as his fingers interlace and squeeze. He leans forward, touching his forehead to mine until the plastic rims of our sunglasses click.

"It's okay," I say, but the truth trickles down my cheeks, collecting at the corners of my mouth. When he presses his lips to mine, the kiss is soft, tentative as if his lips are as bruised as his pride. When our tongues meet they are thick, briny. His is coated with remorse, mine with fear. They tangle, both of them searching for forgiveness.

By the time I get to the bottom of my third beer, I am starting to find some.

"She seduced you right in front of me," I say. He knows exactly who I am talking about.

"You're right," he says.

"The gall of that bitch," I say as I finish my beer and throw the can in the pile of empties at our feet. "Ya know, I've come to terms with you choosing the river over me and going off for six weeks every spring." I stand and cross my arms over my chest. "But you've never before chosen her over me when all three of us are together."

There is silence.

"I guess now that we're on to her, we don't have to worry about that ever happening again, do we?'

"It won't," he says.

I turn and walk through the hot sand on rubbery legs towards the cooler. "Ready for another?" I call over my shoulder. He doesn't answer, but I hear a forceful clang as he hurls his empty one on the pile. By the time we cook dinner, we are laughing hysterically in the dark as we create an off-the-menu meal of Mexican leftovers. After much deliberation, we decide to call it upside down tacos. We eat ravenously, a small mountain of empty beer cans at our feet.

* * *

When I open my eyes the next morning, he is already awake beside me. I see his hand move below our joined sleeping bags.

"Flipping a raft does funny things to me."

I see right through him. It's one of the silly games we play: he tries to trick me into looking at his erection. In the early years, he used to get me all the time. One of the best was, "Whoa, what is *that?*" I yanked my knees up to my breasts, thinking there was a scorpion crawling in our bed. He smiled victoriously and ripped off the covers to reveal his hard cock. But now I recognize the tone to his voice and the slight furrow in his brow when he is trying to come up with something clever.

We've both been riding the emotional highs and lows of feeling horrible and trying to be okay with the fact that we flipped our raft in the Grand Canyon. Right now he is aroused, rested and making light of it. Right now, before caffeine and after dreams of not being able to breathe, I'm not.

"You got the queen wet," I say and roll away from him.

He presses his body into the back of mine and caresses my thigh. "Do I get beheaded for that?" He asks as he kisses my ear, my neck, my shoulder. I don't want his tenderness and curl tighter into myself like a caterpillar.

His calloused hand moves in long, slow strokes across my hips and back with such sweetness that despite myself I feel my body start to relax. He guides me to my back and slides on top of me. With his dark hair, ten-day beard and lithe, athletic body, I feel like I've been pinned by a black panther. He positions his erection against my folds that are as dry and tacky as my tongue and holds me with his gaze. I wish I had my shades to hide the resentment that is still clinging to my eyes like crusty sleep in the corners. I improvise with my eyelids and look down and end up staring right at his river talisman, the piece of jade he wears from the Salmon River. I reach up and slide it around to the back of his neck, out of view.

"It's not fair. You chose the hard line and I got spanked," I say to his Adam's apple.

He takes my hand and puts it on the hard mound of one of his butt cheeks.

"Take your best shot."

I don't hesitate, wind up and slap. "One..." It stings my palm, but I don't care.

He grimaces. "Owww." My adventurer has no problem inflicting incredible amounts of pain on his own body, but he's a total wimp when someone else is doing it.

"Two..." The heat of my slap conducts through his buttock to the tip of his erection that is nudging up against my clit. I feel my folds beginning to melt.

"One more," he closes his eyes and clenches his jaw.

"I get ten," I say.

"Ten?" I feel his gluts tighten under my palm.

I put both of my hands in front of his face, palms open. "Ten."

He places his palm against one of mine and interlaces our fingers. "Hey, I got spanked, too. My guide pride took a beating for one and ...well, those ten seconds you were under...they were the longest ten seconds of my life."

My anger is dissolving, transmuting.

"You get five," he braces himself for the pain. "Three more."

I use both hands. "Three, four, five," I say, slapping his buns like a bongo before gripping the hot flesh of his cheeks and rocking his cock deeper into my clit.

He shakes his head, ridding himself of the pain like a dog shedding water after a bath. "Better?" he asks.

"Wetter." The anger has dissolved, but it has left in its wake the emotion that was driving it all along.

"I don't want to get back on the river," I whisper into his collarbone. We are on day eleven of a twenty-four day trip. There are still 188 miles of river and more black diamond rapids, including the notorious Lava Falls, waiting downstream. "I'm scared."

He cradles my head in his hands and lowers his forehead to mine.

"I won't let anything happen to you." His kisses fall light as mist on my parched lips. "We'll take the easy lines." His tongue seeps between my lips, watering mine. He knows I'm a sucker for his slow, silky kisses. The intensity and passion he brings to whitewater, is now directed at me and by the time his lips drift down my neck and lightly land on my nipple, I am arching my back, pushing my breast deeper into his face.

My knight is poised above me. His jade has somehow worked its way back to the front and it dangles between us, the presentation so obvious, like a queen extending the ring on her hand for me to kiss. His hand drops and circles his tip against my slick bud and the sensation is so exquisite it takes my breath away. But my breath is right there when I want it back, filling my lungs. I realize that the river did, after all, let me go and my knight was right there to rescue me when she did.

The waning moon that has been following us down the river is setting behind my lover's head. As the dawn paints the striated rock of the canyon's north rim in hues of amber and rose, I too, feel lightened. I am deep within one of the earth's most magnificent palaces with a hard-bodied knight lying on top of me, loving me. I bow my head and kiss the smooth green stone as I push my hips forward, impaling myself on my knight's scepter. I lie back, open my arms like wings and surrender.

As my lover thrusts slowly, rhythmically inside me, his jade follows: rocking back and forth, hypnotically, in front of my face. I become entranced by the movement and suddenly I feel her, like a cresting wave moving up my body. She curls, pushing me sideways and I roll, pinning my knight beneath me. I lodge the heel of my hand on his sternum, thread the leather cord of his jade between my fingers and begin to extract my pleasure, grinding wildly into his pubic bone as his scepter bludgeons up against my cervix.

"Rock me," I demand in a voice that I don't recognize as my own, a voice that sounds as if it is scratching its way out of my larynx. His hands move to my hips increasing the intensity of my thrusts. The friction is burning, igniting my clit, flickering heat into my core. My hand grabs one of his and moves it to my ass.

"Give me the other five," I command.

The singe of his slap fuels my fire and I release a haughty laugh, a queen's laugh.

He slaps again, harder this time, and the sting soars like a flaming arrow up my spine and sears across my chest. He bongos out the last three and I am launched, exploding like a geyser into a higher realm of carnal knowledge.

I am bone, blood, breath.

I am water.

CHAPTER EIGHTEEN

May 2008
Lava

I PLANNED TO SKIP WRITING about our experience at Lava Falls, the largest, most anticipated rapid on the Grand Canyon. We didn't have any notably great sex there because I was so unraveled by the roar of the rapid.

Somehow my guide talked me into a layover day at the camp named Above Lava. That means we spent two nights camped right above that monster of a rapid.

Nobody does this. No one would subject their nerves to that kind of torture especially if they had already been spanked by Lava's twin sister Crystal. That is part of the reason my guide suggested a layover there; he knew I was probably the only person he could ever persuade to do it. The other reason was a six-hour hike up to the rim and Vulcan's Throne, the dormant volcano that created Lava Falls and the foreboding black rock that distinguishes that part of the canyon.

I agreed, reluctantly, to the layover/hike option when he agreed, reluctantly, that I could walk the rapid if I wanted. I thought if my psyche knew I had the option to skip the rapid, I could relax, enjoy the hike and the two days camped above it.

My ego thought otherwise.

Walk Lava? Are you some kind of pussy? This, while I'm clawing my way up steep scree at the break of dawn so we can hike the volcano and be back in camp before the mid-day heat of the May desert sun.

"What is so wrong with being a pussy?" I shot back. "What would all you rock-hard cocks do without any pussies around?" It was a good comeback, albeit a strange one, since I was one-upping myself out loud as I climbed. But it was effective, and shut my ego up long enough for me to scramble my way up to the rim.

I'd never been to the Grand Canyon before this trip, so I'd never seen the view from the top looking down. It was stunning, of course, but the best part was being on top of the canyon and hiking under an enormous blue sky on a volcano covered with spring wildflowers. No, actually, the best part was being away from the river. From the rim, she looked like a faraway, insignificant snake.

It wasn't until we started our descent that my ego rallied from behind and scored its winning point.

You mean to tell me that you are willing to look at the picture in Pete's bathroom for the rest of your life knowing that you wimped out and walked Lava?

The answer was no.

We stay with our friend Pete, who lives an hour away from our cabin in a swanky ski town, all the time. By the light switch in the bathroom is a picture of what looks like a raft, and what could be a person, completely engulfed in whitewater. On the bottom, written on the matting are two words: Lava Falls. I couldn't face that picture and my own cowardice for the rest of my life.

I had to run Lava.

True to his word, my guide played it safe. We packed up our camp the next morning and waited, and waited, and waited for another group to come along.

The anticipation was killing me. "Maybe we should just run it on our own and get it over with."

"We will wait."

Within ten minutes a posse of yellow rafts appeared upstream. Turns out they were from the Grand Canyon Institute and their head guide was on his 130th trip down the canyon. They graciously invited us to scout and run the rapid with them.

My guide conferred with theirs as a group of us stood on shore above Lava and scouted the rapid.

"We're going to follow that bubble line above and right of the ledge hole." He pointed down at the river and the massive violent hydraulic that gives Lava its reputation as a bad-ass rapid. "Instinctively, you're going to want to drift off of it as we get close to the hole. Don't."

My whole body trembled as I went to untie our raft. As my guide took the rope from my shaky hands, I noticed balloons tied to one of the yellow rafts parked next to ours. One of the Institute's clients was celebrating his seventieth birthday. He wasn't walking the rapid.

I took my place in the back of the raft, held on tight and kept reminding myself of what I had read in the guidebook. *It takes twenty-three seconds.* It couldn't be any worse than the forty-eight-hour build-up.

We followed the line of the head guide, got unbelievably close to the ledge hole and greased the rapid. We even got some amazing photos e-mailed to us from one of the guides who took photos from the shore before he ran the rapid. He was the one who from then on referred to us as Glen and Bessie.

There's one photo that all you can see beneath a massive wave of whitewater is a hint of dark hair on the oars and a blond braid behind it. I really need to print that one and hang it on the wall in Pete's bathroom.

CHAPTER NINETEEN

May 2008
Rock Hard

THE RED IMPRINT OF MY lover's hand faded from my ass within minutes after my royal spanking. But nine days later, the river's spanking still stings. We've traveled one hundred miles of river without incident since my tryst with Crystal, yet every time the river begins to whiten and froth, despite my yogic breathing and *May we be safe* mantra, my hands begins to shake.

I fear I am becoming my paternal grandmother. Don't get me wrong—Kathleen was loving and sweet. I remember her pulling me into her soft ample breasts, the skin of her face as thin as tissue paper and as soft as velvet against my cheek.

But unlike my mother, who stayed sane raising seven kids with the mantra *No news is good news*, Kathleen worried. All the time. She fretted so much that her whole body trembled. I remember the rattle of her china cup against the saucer as her shaking hand lifted a cup of coffee to her lips, the trembling radiating all the way up to her halo of fine gray hair.

Kathleen's blood runs through my veins. And it's been pulsing through them before every rapid since Crystal. Even though my mom is the rock solid matriarch of my genetic makeup, she also passed along her hypoglycemia. So even if I can keep Kathleen calm, my hands still shake if I don't eat every three hours. I don't have any other female relatives to blame for my endorphin addiction that leaves my biceps quivering after a turn on the oars or that causes my calves to twitch from hiking side canyons. I had my first experience of sewing machine legs, a phenomenon known to climbers, when I followed my guide's lead and found my body stretched between two narrow canyon walls fifteen feet above a stagnant pool of water at Silver Grotto. Halfway across, my legs fatigued and starting pumping out of control as if they could stitch my resolve back together.

So despite how much I'd like to consider myself a fearless chick who can stand next to my man and calmly scout a raft-eating rapid, the reality is this:

It's my legacy to shake. And I hate it.

But right now we are off the river for the day, on solid ground, surrounded by striated red canyon walls as we hike up Parashant Wash. This is an easy hike without any strenuous climbing moves. I'm fed. There is no turbulent water here to make my hands tremble. But there once was. Whatever torrent moved all these rocks and created this wash has been reduced at this time of year to a gentle, lyrical trickle that seeps down the canyon walls, watering all the wildflowers. We're hiking through smooth, rounded rocks of every size imaginable, some as big as a Volkswagen Bug. The narrow walls of this side canyon block out the late afternoon sun, and we are warmed by the heat radiating off the rocks that absorbed the desert sun all day.

Our clothes drop from our bodies as if the seams holding them together have suddenly dissolved. We leave them in a pile with our hats and sunglasses that we no longer need in this ambient shade. We continue hiking, completely comfortable in nothing but our Chaco sandals. We pulled off the river late in the day and made camp at the only access to this wash from the river. We have this shady, radiant rocky canyon garnished with wildflowers, all to ourselves. I feel like we've stepped into Eden. But there are no snakes hanging from the branches of apples trees to tempt me; no wily river mistress waiting to seduce my man.

My C-cup breasts feel surprisingly light and firm without the support of my halter bikini top. We've been rowing, hiking and throwing heavy, metal ammunition cans of food and supplies on and off the raft for the past nineteen days. Our bodies are lean and strong. Our skin is bronzed from the sun and cast in the red earth silt of the canyon. After nearly three weeks of rowing, washing, drinking and sleeping with the river, we are infiltrated and melding into her like natives.

I watch two butterflies land on a bouquet of wildflowers growing out from a crevice in the canyon wall. I feel tranquil to my toes.

I level my hand in front of my face, checking my barometer.

My guide stops and watches me.

"What's the reading?"

My hand hangs still in the air. "Rock steady."

We've safely navigated all the hard rapids of the canyon, including the notorious Lava Falls. I have nothing left to fear. I survived. My marriage survived. Kathleen can finally relax. I lift my hand and my guide high-fives it.

He takes my hand, kisses it and interlaces our fingers as we continue navigating through the wash. He spots a flat rock the size of a king-size bed and guides me there. We lie down, like lizards, absorbing the heat into our backs, and rest. We have everything we need and nothing we don't. I feel a deep, contented peace.

My lover's hand reaches over and rests on my thigh, a sweet simple gesture connecting us. I roll on my side, rest my head on his chest and cross my top leg over his. His arm wraps around my torso and caresses my hip as his lips press against my forehead. Much like we transitioned into nakedness at the beginning of this hike, we move into lovemaking without much thought. When his hand slips between my thighs, my sheath trickles like the canyon walls, watering my flower. I lie flat on my back, opening myself to his touch and the caress of the warm breeze across my breasts. After so much time together, I feel a seamlessness with my lover and this canyon. But not with this rock. Even though it is flat and warm, it is hard. I sit up, lifting the weight of us off my spine and take my turn as guide. I take my lover's hand and lead him to a nearby Volkswagen rock. I lean my belly and breasts up against the warm curve of the boulder. He leans into me from behind.

My belly is soft against the rock. His erection is hard against my folds. I guide him in. We exhale, melding into each other and the warmth of the boulder. This act is as old as our species, this rock even older. As my arms slide up over my head and my chest flattens against it, I wonder what crazy monsoon storm or earth-quaking event prompted this huge, rounded piece of earth to thunder its way down to rest here.

In contrast to the river, this rock feels so solid. We have rowed through layers of geology with exotic names such as Muav Limestone, Tapeats Sandstones, Zoroaster Granite and my favorite to roll around the tongue, Vishnu Schist. I've been so scared at times, so exhausted and so intimidated by the river. Being immersed in the earthy paradise of Parashant, melting into the warmth of this huge rock as my husband melts inside of me, feels like my big reward.

We don't move, savoring the stillness. From this deep pool of contentedness, I feel a flutter at my cervix like the leaves above us that are rattling in the breeze like rice paper castanets. I giggle from the pure sweetness of the sensation. My man feels it, enjoys it with me and nuzzles my neck before he thrusts slowly, once. When he nudges against it, the flutter intensifies, replaced by a tremor that feels like a memory, like the ancient turbulence that moved this boulder to this very spot is echoing back through time and pulsing into my pubic bone.

The sewing machine legs are suddenly back, the hard muscles of my legs weak and trembling. I inhale in an attempt to send some oxygen to my quads, and end up gasping. I lean heavier into the boulder for balance which channels even more of this rock's history into my body.

I feel a surge of panic. I'm losing control.

But then I have a split second awareness that control is just fear in a different dress so I cast it aside like a stripper and open myself to it all: this rock, this canyon, this river, this man, and allow all the emotion, all the intensity of the past nineteen days to erupt from my core. The floor of my pelvis begins to shift like tectonic plates. My root chakra is quaking so hard I swear I would register an eight on the Richter scale. The seismic intensity radiates out from my epicenter to every nerve fiber in my body and I am suddenly rendered so ecstatic, so weak, I can no longer stand. My man's arms wrap around me, supporting me, allowing me to surrender fully to this earth-rocking, full-body orgasm. As his climax crashes into mine, we lose our balance and teeter backwards, laughing and gasping until we come to rest against another rock. The echo of our orgasmic hysteria reverberates off the canyon walls like aftershocks.

Leaning back against my man, slick with sweat and the juice of our ecstasy, I realize that perhaps my legacy to shake isn't so bad after all.

CHAPTER TWENTY

September 2008
Fourth Honeymoon

THERE ARE TWO THINGS I do about once a year for completely different reasons. One I like too much; the other I'm not sure I like at all. I find myself doing both, simultaneously, on the last night of our fourth honeymoon.

In the days leading up to our anniversary, we actually considered breaking Rule #11. We sat on the deck as we took a break from processing elk, and batted around the idea of skipping our annual honeymoon trip down the Green River in Utah.

We'd already done two river trips together, five days on the Rogue River in Southern Oregon and twenty-four days on the Grand Canyon. My lover taught kayaking on the Salmon and guided rafts on the Arkansas and Colorado all summer. It had been an epic river season and we were both pretty saturated. The lodge pole pines were red, dead from the pine beetle epidemic spreading across Colorado so we had dead trees to cut, firewood to split and most importantly to my hunter, another elk, deer and antelope tag to fill.

Our practical selves almost had our hedonists convinced. My scientist had recently landed a full-time wildlife biologist job in Oregon so our days at the cabin were numbered and the aspen were just starting to transform into shimmering gold coins. We didn't know how the hunting was going to be in the Northwest so it made sense to stock up on meat. Once again, a freezer full of wild game was threatening to take precedence over a romantic river trip.

But then we put the decision up to our favorite litmus test: What are we going to remember when we are ninety? Cutting wood and butchering game? Or our fourth, and perhaps last, honeymoon down the Green River? We dropped the bloody knives, threw the chain saw in the shed and started digging out the swim suits and river gear.

We learned our lesson on Honeymoon #3 and had already secured a permit for mid-September, therefore reducing the chance of unseasonably early snowstorms. The strategy worked. We launched on a sunny windless day and paddled the initial twenty-six miles of flat water in record time. Like our maiden voyage down this river on Honeymoon #1, we lounged around naked at beach camps, sipped champagne and sucked fresh mangos off each other. We slept in at Lion Hollow to wait out a small storm and made mountain-lion love to the gentle sound of rain on our tarp.

Even though we'd already eaten the upside down tacos, we saved the most defining elements of Mexican night, the margaritas, for our last night on the river. After a long day of paddling, we ran Rattlesnake rapid and were thrilled to see the camp below it of the same name, deserted, waiting for a couple of hedonists to settle in for the night.

Rattlesnake is one of our favorite camps, with a long flat beach by the river and a wind-protected camp tucked up in the tamarisk. It had the extra bonus of Rattlesnake Canyon a short hike from camp that was perfect for trail-running in September. On Honeymoon #3 we followed bear tracks up the soft, muddy creek bed. This year we ran into a herd of bighorn sheep. Afterward, we bathed in the warmth of the afternoon sun and pulled out our last clean shirts that we'd been saving for our party—a Hawaiian shirt for him and a floral thrift store find for me. We sat on the beach sipping margaritas as the sun cast the canyon walls in pink.

As the tequila penetrated our parched, sun-drenched bodies, our inner teenagers, who grew up in the era of beer bongs and quarters, emerged and organized a drinking game with our forty-something fitness freaks. This involved sprinting from the river up a steep, sandy hill to the edge of the tamarisk, taking a sip of margarita and then racing back down to the river. Twice. He beat me all three times before we realized that the sun had set and we needed dinner. As he built a fire on the beach, I threw together a plate of our remaining food that gratefully required no cooking: slices of cheese, dried sausage, apples, mustard and crackers. For dessert I refilled the platter with orange slices and dark chocolate, and grabbed the remnants of a bottle of red wine leftover from Italian night. The sight of those squares of dark chocolate softening on the plate next to the fire ignited one of my deepest desires.

"I'm thinking of breaking the moratorium on chocolate tonight." I tried to sound casual and in control as I began to fondle the chocolate bar, breaking off more little squares and arranging them on the plate.

His expression changed from surprise to concern. He, more than anyone, knows what chocolate does to me. I get wired and giddy for about two hours and then crash into an irritable, irrational heap. And then, I want more. I swore off of it right after our wedding, determined not to bring my chocoholism into our marriage. He humors me and puts up with me smelling his brownies and French-kissing him right after he takes a bite of chocolate cake. Except for a handful of lapses, I haven't really had chocolate in four years.

"Uh….are you sure about that?" He was trying really hard to be the rational one.

"Well, this is a very special occasion—the last night of our last Green River honeymoon. For a while anyway." We've both started adding the 'for a while' phrase because we were still in denial of the implications of a full-time biologist job eight hundred miles from this river. "I mean, really…what am I going to remember when I'm ninety? Eating a few orange slices or rubbing this chocolate all over your cock and licking it off?"

Within seconds, he stands naked in front of me, holding the desert plate in front of my face.

My clothes land in a heap in the sand on top of his. Our bonfire is raging now, an entity in itself, fiery arms dancing and reaching out to warm our bare skin.

I take a piece of chocolate and run it down the length of his erect cock, painting him in wide stripes like a skunk. I follow the lines with the entire width of my tongue, slowly at first, savoring, giving into a craving that I've been managing for years. But once my desire is unleashed, I lick, suck and practically swallow him whole, devouring the bittersweet taste of my two most favorite addictions.

My lust for his chocolate cock is so vigorous that it isn't long before I get a 'ding'. I pull back and give him a couple seconds to regain control while I take a sip of red wine, the perfect complement to my dark chocolate cock dessert. When I dive back in, I get a few more dings but I'm not interested in reciprocation. Just chocolate. I can feel its dark stickiness all over my face, making strands of hair stick to my cheek. A crazed giggle bubbles up my throat as I grab another square and begin to paint him in curlicue waves that swirl around his testicles. My eyes roll back in ecstasy as my tongue sways and circles between his thighs, licking until he is glistening and clean. I reach for another square, ready to paint him with stars, when he grabs my sticky fingers, brings them to his lips and kisses them.

"You'll thank me in the morning," he says as he drops to his knees. He guides my hand away from my own destruction and turns my body away from the platter.

The smell of burning driftwood fills my nostrils. The heat of the fire warms my low back as he guides me down on my hands and knees. He lies beneath me and kisses my labia and breasts that are hanging above him like ripe fruit from a tree. He caresses my haunches and litters soft kisses inside my thighs. I sense his desire for something different just as his fingers, slippery with saliva, moisten my super sensitive sphincter. This is usually when I giggle and jump away but I am so relaxed, so euphoric and satiated that instead, I push into his hand. He continues his gentle exploration there as his other hand strokes my clit. The kisses that brush across my low back are so tender, so encouraging. I lick the remnants of dark chocolate from my lips. The taste is sweet like his kisses; bitter like the idea of his cock pushing into my tight rectum, a sensation that is so intense that I'm not sure if I like it or hate it. But it is a night to do things I don't normally do, a moment in our marriage that we will never have again. The last night of what could be our last honeymoon on the Green River.

The bottle of lube is like the camera, packed somewhere in our dry bags and never around when we need it. My lover is nothing if not resourceful. As he mounts me from behind, he takes advantage of the wetness that is already there and slides his cock into my slick sheath. This, I know I like. I push back into him and we thrust, mountain lion style, as he nuzzles my neck and growls, bringing me up to a quivering climax. He pulls out and allows himself a partial release, spreading his warm lube like melted butter across my tight hole. His touch is soft again, gentle, as he pushes slowly in.

The sensation burns like a shot of tequila, like the embers of the fire glowing beside me. He moves slowly, inching deeper and then back in a small range of motion gauging my gasps, both of us breathing raggedly with this hot, tight intensity.

I hit my limit a second before he does and suddenly the pain overrides any sense of pleasure and I move forward and away. My entire spine shivers from the expulsion and I savor the light tingling left behind. I descend, panting, to my forearms and release a shaky sigh. I look over my shoulder at the fiery silhouette of my lover as he slides his hand down his shaft once, twice. His orgasm flows like warm lava on my lower back.

We are a chocolate-sticky mess. He stands and guides me to the river where we wash in the dark water, laughing and howling like a couple of coyotes. We settle back in next to the fire, a large towel wrapped around us as we huddle close to dry.

Gazing into the fire, I have a moment where it seems like I am hovering, watching us from above, as if the lens of my memory is panning back. I see us, a primal tangle of limbs illuminated by the orange hue of firelight, the only color on the river on this new moon night. I see our tanned bodies entwined in passion, surrounded by canyon walls that radiate the warmth of the September sun well past midnight. I see the Milky Way, like spilled glitter, sparkling above us.

Remember this, I think. And I will, when I am ninety, holding hands with my husband as we sit beside a roaring fire, sipping red wine and eating chocolate. As we warm our worn joints, we will relive that night when we got down and dirty on all fours in the sand by the river. The image will sustain us in those dimming years, when memory is our greatest lover.

CHAPTER TWENTY-ONE

November 2008
Coming Home

I AM DRIVING WEST on Highway 84 towards the Oregon border. Eleven hours ago when I started this journey, my I-pod froze up as solid as the ice on the Wyoming highway. I've been working the scan button on the radio ever since. Knowing I will surely die if I hear another Billy Joel song or more coverage on the auto industry bailout, I turn it off.

Even though I am alone, it is anything but quiet in the cab of this seventeen-foot-long U-Haul truck. I am accompanied by the cacophony of thoughts that travel with a woman in transition. As I drive past fields brown from November, a line from a 70's song, much like those I was subjected to as I drove through Utah, rises like the sun from the dull incessant chatter inside my head.

I'm coming home to a place I've never been before.

As I cross into Eastern Oregon, I'm amazed that John Denver of all people could sum up my life right now. Punchy from not enough sleep and too much gas station coffee, I launch into the song's chorus and realize that after twenty-five years, my Colorado Rocky Mountain High is officially over. My home is in Northeast Oregon now, a place I've never been.

The last time I moved across the country, I was eighteen and traveling light. Under the guise of a college education, I left my family home in Northern Michigan for the mountains of Colorado with a pair of skis, a ten-speed bike and two duffle bags. Although that first semester at college I missed the fiery, red-maple autumn, the fresh apple cider and the Lake Michigan salmon, Colorado's fall had its own gifts with gold-coin aspen leaves, roasted green chilies and a seemingly endless Indian summer. But it was the record-breaking snowfall that winter that sealed my fate as a Coloradoan. It's a good thing the devil wasn't around searching for souls because I would have willingly traded mine for the continued ecstasy of skiing through waist-deep powder on blue-sky winter days. It wasn't, as John would say, almost heaven. It was the real thing. I had found my home.

But home, as they say, is where the heart is and mine now beats in cadence with my wildlife biologist who left Colorado five weeks ago for a research biologist position with the Oregon Department of Fish and Wildlife. He's been in Port Townsend, Washington, this week, learning how to safely administer drugs used to sedate the cougars he will be collaring and studying in the Blue Mountains. We are currently driving towards each other for a passionate reunion at the rental home he found for us in La Grande.

I push my foot harder down on the accelerator as I think of how close I am to seeing his ruggedly, handsome face and notice a sign indicating that I am on the forty-fifth parallel, half way between the North Pole and the equator. I recognize that sign and realize it is the same one posted on the highway by my childhood home in Northern Michigan. The thought of returning to that long ago latitude makes me smile.

Off the interstate I begin to notice closed fruit stands and orchards with a few apples still weighing heavily on the branches. I've been living at 8,000 feet for the past fourteen years and the idea of living in a fruit-growing region with fresh apple cider again sends a rush of enthusiasm through my road-weary body. As I pass through Baker City, I am warmed by the snow-capped mountains forming the backdrop to the town.

As a casual student of Buddhism, I've often aspired towards the idea of the Middle Path. When the highway winds downhill, I shift the truck into low gear and wonder if perhaps I'm getting close since I seem to be in the middle of many things. The northern hemisphere, for one. At forty-three, I'm somewhere, hopefully, in the middle of my life. And this new home in Eastern Oregon with its orchards *and* mountains seems to be mid-way between the ones I have known in Michigan and Colorado.

I follow my husband's directions and take the first La Grande exit that takes me through the center of town. We aren't being facetious when we jokingly refer to our new town as 'The Big' because it *is* big compared to the isolated mountain hamlet of six hundred people where we had been living in Colorado. I marvel at how authentic it looks here with a J.C. Penney store, non-franchised restaurants and an old movie theatre with the name, *The Granada,* spelled out in a vintage script above the marquee. I turn onto First Street and see towering evergreens and hardwood trees beside charming homes still decorated with pumpkins and scarecrows. Children are laughing and playing in piles of dried leaves while their parents rake.

I barely have the truck in park as I jump out at the blue and white house with the address my husband gave me. I'm the first to arrive and find the key where he stashed it for me under the welcome mat. The house is cold when I step inside the kitchen, but as I round the corner into the living room, sunlight floods in the south-facing windows. I find the thermostat left at fifty-five degrees and inch it up. In the bedroom, I see his hiking boots and his favorite brown and white wool sweater from Chili by the bed. Exhilarated to finally be here but exhausted from the drive, I pull off my wrinkled, travel-weary clothes and climb naked under the autumn-colored quilt his mother made for us. I bury my head in his pillow and breathe in his rumpled head-hair scent.

I am home.

I awake to the sound of a creaking door followed by footsteps on linoleum. I open my eyes just in time to see his body flying, arms spread wide like a superhero, from the foot of the bed towards me. He lands on top of me and his mouth, like a heat-seeking missile, finds mine. I always forget how juicy and moist his lips are, as I hope he forgets the dry, tacky quality of mine. He saturates my lips as his hands auger under the covers searching for the rest of me. His calloused hands, like fine sandpaper, explore my curves, turning the past five weeks of longing to dust. Now that he is on top of me, it feels like we've never been apart. The angles of his face, the smell of his breath, the weight of him are all so familiar. But there is a freshness to him, to us, like worn sheets that have dried outside on a summer day.

My body is so hungry for his touch that when his hand slides from my breast to my folds, they are already salivating. This is the antithesis of a Farewell Fuck when we linger and savor every detail of each other. In a Reuniting Fuck, we gorge. There is so much sensation, so much pleasure in what is usually our standard foreplay. Just the thought of his body penetrating mine makes my cervix quiver.

His tip nudges against my opening. Our eyes lock. Our lips touch. Our mouths stretch into simultaneous smiles. We release mutual sighs—of relief, of completion—as he glides into me.

Missionary position has never felt so good. I want nothing less than full genital to genital contact, our hearts thumping into each other's chests, the brown of his iris swirling into my blue. All the longing and mental grasping of the last few weeks shifts to the physical realm. My hands reach around and squeeze the firm flesh of his gluts before wrapping around his waist. My core tightens. My sheath hugs his cock in the deepest embrace.

Our bodies, like our lives now, are fully melded. We have one home, one car, one phone, one bed.

I've never before, in the four years since our wedding, felt so married.

CHAPTER TWENTY-TWO

January 2009
Mounting Emily

WHEN WE MOVED TO OREGON, my backcountry skier didn't waste any time finding a new winter mistress.

And right now I hate them both.

I was so easily seduced by this new girl. Our first month in Oregon, the state was hit with unseasonably cold, snowy weather. Every time we ventured out to explore Mount Emily, the low-elevation peak just fifteen minutes (by car!) from our rental house, we discovered waist-deep, fluffy snow on low-angled slopes with no threat of avalanche. I thought he had finally found a sweet mistress, all champagne and silk, one that wasn't lying in wait for an opportunity to bring me to my knees.

But today, five hours into a mission to reach a new aspect of her face that we haven't skied yet, she pulled out the leather and whips. The snow that landed like angel kisses on my nose this morning is now sleet that is coming down sideways and pelting my face like tiny arrows. The foot of fresh powder that brushed our shins as we kicked and glided from the parking lot is now eight inches of wet cement mortared to the bottom of my skis. The short arc of the winter sun is dipping towards the horizon and we still have five miles of uphill climbing to get to the trailhead where our truck is parked. Each step (my skis quit gliding hours ago) hurts. I've been following him up this mountain like an excited puppy for the past two weeks, trying to gobble up this storm that shut down Portland and now my hip flexors and quads are the ones shutting down. I'm on that adventure precipice where I feel so tired and defeated that I want to cry.

And my man, whose Southern upbringing leaks out every now and then, is whistling *Dixie*. He thrives on this, the more miserable the better. I feel like a beleaguered soldier lagging behind some crazed general.

The worst part is I have no one to blame but my various selves. I woke up this morning fully intending to stay home. The few people we'd met in La Grande kept telling us that this winter was unseasonably cold and snowy; that it would soon get warm and melt the snow. They said this because they thought it was what we wanted to hear. Instead, they threw us into a panic, triggering the most fanatical depths of our ski bum souls. We'd been gobbling up powder for the past two weeks and I was full, painfully so.

"I'm going to take a rest day," I said as we sat across from each other on the couch, legs entangled, sipping coffee. He nodded, an outward attempt at support, and said nothing. I was surprised he was letting me off so easily.

But he wasn't letting me off at all. He was just waiting until the caffeine was in my system before he delivered his pitch.

"I'm going for The Virgins today, could be the last day to try. It's supposed to rain tonight."

My man knows my buttons and just how to push them. The first slope we discovered on Mt. Emily was the most obvious, one the locals call Cloud Nine. The next week we followed some tracks to a run we dubbed Seventh Heaven. From there we eyed a new aspect of Emily's face that we've been fantasizing about skiing ever since. Keeping with the theme, we've been referring to this one as The Fourteen Virgins after the Islamic extremist belief that heaven, for those who make the ultimate sacrifice for the cause, like a suicide bomber, get rewarded in the afterlife with fourteen virgins.

And now my backcountry skier is taunting me with them. Today, with rising temperatures predicted, this could be the last window to ski that untouched slope.

My various selves start jostling for power.

The Pathetic Wife: *You can't let him go alone, it's too dangerous! He needs you. You have to go.*

The Tomboy: *Don't let him deflower that beauty without you. Get your lazy ass off the couch and go get dressed. You'll be fine.*

The Teenager: *Get rid of the boy. We can stay right here on the couch all day and eat pizza and tortilla chips and watch movies.*

The Yoga Teacher: *Honor your body's need to rest.*

The Tomboy: *You can rest when you're dead.*

But it's The Writer who pulls out the trump card: *Stay home if you want, but we could use some new material and besides, what are you going to remember when you are ninety?*

I was off the couch in minutes, making a peanut butter and jelly sandwich, organizing my pack.

My backcountry skier yelled from the bedroom, "Don't forget your headlamp." It was barely dawn, not yet 7:30 in the morning. Granted, Oregon days in early January were short, but not that short. I should have known right then. I should have run back to the couch, pulled the afghan over my head, and huddled with my teenager and yoga-teaching selves.

But I didn't. I ignored every wise voice in my head screaming *Rest Day!* and put that damned headlamp in my pack at dawn.

And we didn't even get to The Virgins. By the time we broke trail through miles of deep snow, bushwhacked through thick brambles around an icy creek crossing, and got to the base of the slope, the temperatures had already started warming. All the fresh fluffy new snow had turned heavy enough to slide.

Sure, I was disappointed that we expended so much effort only to get spurned by The Virgins. But, I have to admit, the disappointment was intertwined with the relief of not having to climb another 1,000 feet of vertical and contend with the angst of skiing an unfamiliar, avalanche-prone slope. The relief was short-lived, though, when the reality of getting back set in. We had to break fresh trail, uphill, in heavy snow that clung to our skis like papier-mâché.

My Teenager couldn't help but gloat. *If you had listened to me, me, me, we would be warm and dry on the couch right now, missing all this misery.*

"Shut up," I told her. "Go stuff your face with Doritos." I apologized to the Yoga Teacher and then went searching for the support of the selves that got me into this. The Tomboy wasn't much help. *Dude, like, sorry, I forgot about all the climbing. I was more psyched about the downhill part.*

Desperate, I reached out to The Writer. "You got me into this, please help me out."

She tossed me a memory, like a bone to chew on, as I kept climbing.

We were in Vail staying with my husband's uncle who was vacationing there. I was enjoying getting to know Jim, a handsome man of seventy who was feeling the altitudinal difference between his home in Alabama and the ski runs of Vail Mountain.

"Don't you try and keep up with him," he said as he nodded across the lodge at his nephew who was battling the lunchtime crowds to get the three of us some hot tea. "He's just like my dad who lived to be ninety-eight. He was a powerhouse his whole life. He ate ice cream and bacon and was always thin as a reed and strong as steel. I guess that kind of thing skips a generation," he said as he patted his belly beneath his ski sweater.

I knew at the time I was getting some sage advice. I have no idea why I didn't remember it until now. I mean, really, I am trying to keep pace with a guy that is six-foot, strong as an ox, pumping with testosterone, and even more driven than usual to recreate since he's taken on a full-time job that limits his recreation to two days a week.

Before I met my adventurer, I fantasized about a man with six-pack abs and a rock-hard ass. I know I'm not alone on this one. And finding that has been amazing, don't get me wrong. But those assets don't evolve from hanging out on the couch eating pizza and watching movies on the weekend. There is a reason a man has a hot, hard body. Unless he is twenty or just genetically gifted, he is usually obsessed with some kind of physical activity. If you aren't keen to go with him, you'll spend your weekends alone. If you dig deep and find the courage to accompany him, you'll be pushing your limits ninety percent of the time.

So I know you've heard this before, but I am going to say it again. Be careful what you wish for. I longed for a passionate, sexy, strong, adventurous man. By some stroke of luck, I got him. Right now I am out here with his sleet-pelting mistress, earning it.

When I look at my current situation in that light, rather than the impending darkness of an Oregon January evening, I find the strength to keep going.

CHAPTER TWENTY-THREE

February 2009
Alternative Healing

MY WILDLIFE BIOLOGIST and I are slumped against opposite arms of the couch, facing each other and a gray Sunday morning in Oregon. Rain is pouring down, obliterating any chance of skiing Mt. Emily again this season. We knew we were on borrowed time with our low-elevation, Oregon mistress, but we had no idea our love affair with her would end this soon. We miss Colorado and long to get drunk on Mount Hailey's champagne powder. We are fighting off the same cold. Our spirits are low.

"I need a doctor." I take the last sip of my tea and set the empty cup on the coffee table.

The transformation in him is immediate. His demeanor shifts with his spine as he straightens and sits up.

"The doctor is in." His left brow lifts purposefully as his voice takes on a contrived, compassionate tone. "Tell me, what is bothering you?" His hand begins to caress my ankle.

"I have a sore throat." I pull off his socks and reach for the waistband of his fleece pants and pull them down his legs.

"Hmmm, a sore throat. Well, then, let me see...well... yes, of course. You need throat therapy."

"Throat therapy?" I feign ignorance of his standard remedy for any ailment (including hangnails and shaving nicks) as we pull off each other's sweatshirts.

"Well, of course, nothing else will do. Nothing stimulates healing to the body quite like the rubbing of the cock against the back of the throat." He relieves me of my pink satin pajama bottoms, leaving my mint-green lace thong in place.

"Really?" I lean forward between his legs and rub my nose against his platinum-colored silk boxers. "Are you sure all that rubbing won't make it worse?" I let my hand travel down, exploring the silver silk until I feel his cock twitch and strain against the fabric.

"No, no...of course not." He waves his hand dismissively. "Throat therapy is incredibly healing. I'm a doctor, I know about these things."

"If you say so..." I play along with his cock-against-the-epiglottis theory, because I love his dreamy Dr. of Sexology voice. But it isn't the throat therapy that heals me. My nose pushes into the crease between his upper thigh and scrotum and sniffs like a German shepherd searching for drugs. Nothing yet.

I quickly relieve him of the silk boxers, slide back down between his thighs and trace the tip of my nose along the rugged ridge that dissects his sac. My tongue follows with wide, wet strokes up his shaft. Once he is coated and slick, I proceed with the prescribed therapy, descending on his probe with an open jaw. When his tip nudges up against the tender part of my throat, I swirl it around like a cotton swab testing for strep. My lips circumvent and seal around his base before I drag them slowly up. I repeat this sequence several times, basic throat therapy, he thinks, but really I am priming him like a pump. Fingers interlaced, I work his slick rod between both palms, extracting oil from his well. I auger my nose deep into the warm, mammalian juncture of his thigh and put my yoga training to good use with a deep, bronchiole-filling inhalation.

I suppose most women with a cold would be going for the mentholated, antiviral qualities of eucalyptus right now. Or maybe the relaxing, sleep-inducing qualities of lavender. Hippie girls need nothing but patchouli. My essential oil lies deep beneath the surface of my lover's rock-hard cock.

On an exploratory mission for my ultimate elixir, I kiss and caress his sac with both hands. When he moans, his testicles contract, releasing the scent of his arousal like a couple of perfume atomizers. Wanting to absorb it through every orifice, I burrow my nose, my lips, my tongue into his loins. He smells of musk, yes, but so much more.

My tongue descends, exploring the round contours of his sac and I detect sweetness, reminding me of dark cherries, warm and ripened by the July sun. I imagine them hanging heavy from the branches as I suck his dangling fruit and work the flesh of his sac in my palms.

He moans and I smell autumn: the fertile, dark soil of composted leaves. His scent is rich and abundant, like the harvest; nutty and sweet like butternut squash.

My hair falls forward like a curtain, containing his heat. He smells yeasty, of homemade bread, warm from the oven on a winter afternoon. My hands reach around and knead the hard dough of his gluts.

Keeping up the throat therapy ruse, I let his cock nudge up against the back of my throat again. But it is my nose, lingering above his fur that I am most aware of. When he moans again, my sinuses fill with a pungency that reminds me of my favorite imported Swiss cheese, stimulating an olfactory memory: we are at the cabin eating Gruyere and sipping red wine. I imagine the heady bouquet of a Cabernet evaporating on my tongue as I lick down his shaft and back to his tip. The drop of pre-cum there is salty, like sweat, from a day of skiing Mount Hailey. Salty, like the sweat trickling down my ribcage as the heat of his arousal radiates on my face.

I blow on his hot cock lightly, a spring breeze verdant and fragrant of grass. When he catches his breath, I blow more of mine, pursing my lips and directing its cool stream over both of us. His testicles contract. My nipples stiffen. The chill travels down my spine and floods my sheath like a creek overflowing with the run-off. Spring means strawberries, sticky and sweet on his warm cock. I feel a tremor at my clit as it remembers the sensation of strawberry seeds rubbing against it during one of our more memorable Farewell Fucks.

"Yummmmm..." I let the sound of the 'm' vibrate at the base of his shaft. I'm having an odoriferous orgy here—all four seasons and a picnic–between his thighs. Greedy for more, I slather his shaft with my salivary juices and launch into a frenzy of licking, sucking and pumping.

"Ding. Ding. Ding." His head rocks back and forth, a chasmal smile on his face. He grabs my shoulders and pulls my gluttonous mouth to his.

"Well now, you really are excelling with the throat therapy." He does the voice, the cocky eyebrow thing. "Tell me, how is your throat feeling?"

"My throat?" I swallow. Damn, if it doesn't feel better. But I can't bring myself to feed my arrogant sexologist's ego and tell him. I clear my throat dramatically. "A little better," I say weakly.

This is usually when he starts lecturing about clit therapy and demonstrates the healing effects of cunnilingus. But we both know that is out this morning because of the hint of a cold sore forming on his lip.

"Better, but not gone?" He looks *so* concerned. "Hmmm…we better follow up with some infusion therapy just to make sure."

"Infusion therapy?"

"But of course." Another dismissive wave of the hand. "I infuse you with my super healing fluids. It's a preventative measure. Helps build your immunity. Trust me, I'm a doctor."

He turns me and pulls my back to his chest. "You see, for ailments of the throat, the infusion therapy must be done backwards." He pulls me on his lap and wraps his arms around me. One hand lands on a breast. The other pushes away my thong and rests on my vulva. And then, like a classical guitarist, he begins to strum. My body melts into his and all it takes is a subtle shift of my hips and his healing probe is inside of me.

We lie back and I feel suspended, my back floating on his chest and abdomen that are firm yet fluid from lap swimming. He holds me like a flute now, his fingers playing my nipple and clit as his mouth kisses and nuzzles my neck. Moans of pleasure flow musically from my lips.

My throat therapy has brought him so close, so many times. Now the warmth and tightness of my body bring him up fully. He grips my hips and pulses with short, deep thrusts. His orgasm is right there and the force of it triggers mine. Our backs arch in unison, our chests lift to the sky, our bodies stacked in a simultaneous orgasmic fish pose. We flail, as if we were flung from the sea on to the beach, both of us gasping for breath.

His palm rests on my mons, securing me to him as his fingers continue to play, swirling around on my bud to encourage more tremors. His other hand caresses my hair as he extracts a few strands of it from his mouth.

"Tell me, how are you feeling now?"

I swallow. My throat doesn't hurt at all. My body buzzes with energy. I can't deny it.

"You are such an amazing doctor."

"But of course." His hand leaves my hair and moves emphatically in front of my face as he speaks. "As I said, the throat therapy, followed by an infusion, is incredibly healing."

My hand reaches down and wafts, encouraging our co-mingled scent to drift up our bodies. I complete my aromatherapy session with a deep inhalation of our coitus cologne.

But of course.

CHAPTER TWENTY-FOUR

April 2009
Her Without Him

I'M LYING ALONE IN MY sleeping bag beside the Colorado River at the put-in for the Grand Canyon. Although 'alone' probably isn't the most accurate description. Fifteen other people are tucked into this tall grass camp.

My man isn't one of them.

I hear guitar and a man's voice singing *Wish You Were Here* by Pink Floyd. It's so appropriate.

Tomorrow morning, almost a year to the day from last year, I will launch on my second Grand Canyon raft trip. But this year I will be launching without my river knight. This will be the first time *ever* I will be on a river without him.

I lie beneath the ink-black sky dusted with stars and determine the singer must be Graham. His lover, like mine, is hiking in on Day Eight at Phantom Ranch. My wildlife biologist is presenting some research at a conference in Spokane so he will be arriving late to this party.

Last year's permit was pure luck, a lottery for a cancellation permit. This permit is the result of three Otter Bar kayak instructors putting down their after-work beers and heading to the computer to combine their years on the waiting list. My man has placed me in good hands. I'm with a posse of outdoor adventure professionals from the US and New Zealand.

But lest you think I am some kind of eager river chick, let me be clear about this: I'm not ready to do this trip again. I could have used a few more years between me and Crystal. Back in January when we started making preparations for this trip, I woke up in the middle of the night, my heart racing with anxiety about facing this river and her big churning rapids again so soon.

But two tickets to paradise don't come often. With the Grand Canyon, you go when the permits are available and ours came two years in a row. And the agony of staying in Northeast Oregon with FOMO (Fear Of Missing Out) actually sounded worse than staring down Crystal again.

Furthermore, I refuse to let Kathleen, the part of me that takes after my nervous grandmother, keep me from twenty-one days on the Grand Canyon with fifteen of our river friends and Kiwi Dave (you met him in Chapter Ten) as the trip leader.

I hug my pillow to my chest in my man's absence and wonder what the Queen has in store for me this year.

It doesn't take long to find out.

Every morning I wake before everyone, even the dawn, and watch the stars fade into blue. As the sun rises, I reach for it from Tree pose, my feet rooted in the sand. At night when the rest of the crew sips Maker's Mark around the fire, I slip away to dance with the moon and flirt with the river as I kick my toes through the shallow water at the beach's edge.

I was a little worried what it would be like to be on the river with fifteen people since I'm so accustomed to just two. But no one notices or misses me when I disappear on my own. I've developed a keen sense of locating the guide sites, obscure patches of flattened grass big enough for one, tucked away beside the river. The river's voice is the last thing I hear before I fall asleep and the first thing I hear upon waking.

Interestingly, I find the solitude I've been missing since my man and I moved to Oregon and became so married.

On this upper stretch of the Colorado River that runs through Marble Canyon, there's only one rapid worthy of scouting. The river isn't in vampy mistress mode. Instead, she's the kind of woman lover I would choose, all soft, curvy and sweet-lipped. I find myself entranced with her side canyons and mesmerized by the play of light that heightens the striated color of her geology at sunset.

For a woman like me who hooks into the divine through nature, this place is like the Sistine Chapel. I'm worshipping day and night, slipping into yoga postures as the sun slips in and out of the canyon. By Day Three I'm pulsing with a blissful sexual energy that I continue to churn through my yoga practice since my man isn't around to share it. But I don't feel sexually deprived at all. I feel so incredibly free like I'm suspended in this emotionally orgasmic state.

I often share the morning light with Graham the guitar player, who is also Graham the professional photographer. One morning he takes a few shots of me doing yoga by the river. By the time we get to the confluence of the Little Colorado River, I ditch my bikini in the sand and ask him to capture me naked in the warm turquoise water.

I think of my man but I'm so enchanted with the river that I don't really miss him. I remember the early years of our relationship when we were so desperately in love and eager to be together and how confusing it was that he could so easily leave me for six weeks to go kayak the Salmon River.

I totally get it now.

CHAPTER TWENTY-FIVE

May 2009
Courting Crystal

MY RIVER KNIGHT IS BACK on the oars as we head into the Inner Gorge of the Grand Canyon. I am perched above and behind him on my upside-down-kayak-of-a-throne, not feeling one bit like a queen.

The rest of our sixteen-person crew is on alert, cautiously moving towards some of the biggest rapids we've seen so far on this trip.

Not my man. He hasn't even had the last eight days to warm up, yet his twenty-something-raft-guide self is cracking a beer before noon when big rapids like Granite, Grapevine and Crystal await us.

At the first rapid, he purposely rows right into the beef of the whitewater, and I get hit, like a slap in the face, with a cold, soaking splash from the river. It's a rude awakening since my previous oarsman, Chris, took extra care since he wanted to deliver his buddy's wife in one piece.

Within thirty minutes of being on the oars, the river's seduction is in full swing and it feels like my man is choosing her over me again, just like last year.

Our plan today is to run the Inner Gorge past Crystal and have a layover day. I'm a bit on edge, to say the least, knowing I have to face that rapid at the end of the day. My man, however, is over the edge with excitement celebrating the first day of his vacation with all his river friends in his favorite place in the world. He's having a second and then a third beer when we stop for lunch.

I confide in our friend Bugs, who spent her twenties raft-guiding with my man and her thirties competing on the Women's National

Whitewater Team. She's a big fan of these river erotica stories and has heard many of them over the kitchen table at the cabin.

"Bugsy, help me out," I say as we sit and balance turkey sandwiches on our knees at lunch. "He's getting seduced by the river, do you see it?"

"Yeah," she says as she looks across the beach at him downing a Tecate. "Drinking beer before Crystal, I wish I was that confident. But don't worry, Little Peanut, he could run Crystal with his eyes closed."

I haven't read *A Royal Spanking* to her yet so she doesn't know I got spanked by Crystal last year.

"Give him a gentle yogic nudge, you're good at that."

I catch him alone and lead him into the tamarisk and try to be very even-keeled and cool, even though my belly is churning so much I couldn't eat much lunch.

"The last thing I want to do is ruin your fun, but just so you know, the river has your face wedged into her big, fat whitewater cleavage, just like last year. And I'm nervous as hell about running Crystal." My voice quivers as I utter the "C" word which gives my little speech some authenticity.

"We're running Crystal today?" he asks.

"Yes, that's the plan, to camp below Crystal and have a layover day."

"I didn't realize that," he says as he looks at his nearly empty beer can and takes the last sip. "But, no worries, baby." He pulls me into a hug and talks into my hair. "We'll take the easy line, and besides, we have tons of backup this year. It will be fun." He looks down at me and smiles so authentically and deep, like I haven't seen in months. When he kisses me, I feel his carefree joy melt through his lips into mine.

He has a point. If I were to get dethroned this year, one of our three expert kayakers who run every rapid first and wait in the eddies like angels, would snatch me out of the river in seconds.

But Kathleen isn't so easily appeased. I choke down a few chips and wish I could fast-forward through this day.

When we finally pull over to scout Crystal at 4:00, she is huge and churning just like I remember. Everyone is tired and I'm not the only one intimidated by her. Our trip leader decides that we will make our two-day layover camp right above the rapid.

The relief of not having to run Crystal with my man who is fresh on the oars and three beers gone is muddled by the fact that now I have to camp above this monster of a rapid for two nights and listen to her roar. It's like Lava Falls all over again and proof positive that whatever you resist, persists.

That night after dinner I slip sway by myself and hike to a vista above the rapid. A half moon is glowing overhead through a thin cloud layer that gives it a soft, mystical effect like those filters they use on cameras when they film older actors.

The effect on Crystal is the same. In this light, she doesn't feel like some haughty queen that wants to spank me senseless. She looks more like an enchantress encouraging me to hook into that part of myself that showed up here again.

I sit cross–legged in the soft moonlight listening to the percussive of her whitewater. I breathe in deeply and feel the magnificence of this place tingling through the downy hair on my arms.

Or maybe it's just fear.

The next morning someone figures out that it is Sunday and since we are having a layover day, we begin to act like it. We have a big buffet of eggs and Canadian bacon. After breakfast we realize if we weren't laying over, we'd be running Crystal at that very moment so we all hike downstream to take a look. She is sleeping in, dreamy, half the size of yesterday afternoon.

The flows on the river vary depending on how much power they are generating up at the Glen Canyon dam. Less power is needed on the weekends so water flows are lower. Yesterday's Saturday flow is hitting us today which means we will have a low Sunday flow, just like today, when we run it tomorrow.

The realization is like a big-bowed gift. We unknowingly ran Crystal at a high flow last year. I feel myself relax a little and then try to convince Kathleen that the rapid is going to be mellow and sweet tomorrow when we run it. She isn't so easily appeased so I tuck her in the shade and tell her to chill out.

I end up doing yoga on the rafts with some of the women. My man helps erect a shade tarp. We catch each other's eyes across camp but then get pulled into separate group activities. Eventually in the late afternoon, he finds me, grabs my hand and leads me downstream, away from the group to a low-water beach.

He hands me a beer and we strip off our clothes and bathe. After we dry off, he continues to guide.

"Let's go see her." I know he's not talking about Bugs. He slips into his shorts and I wrap my sarong around my torso. We follow a path worn well from scouting.

Now that it is afternoon, Crystal is churning again, wide awake from her morning slumber.

She's all tongue at the top of the rapid, where the smooth glassy water makes its last display. She begins here.

So do we.

I spin as my guide unfurls my sarong. He lays it across a big rock beside the river and leans me back on to it. He slides his shorts down his legs so we are both in nothing but our Chaco sandals.

Our tongues tangle lazily, warm and thick with the taste of beer. His roams down my neck, across my collar bone and descends towards my breasts that he cups in both hands, bringing my nipples closer together so he can lavish his attention on them equally. His attention drops into my cleavage and keeps flowing downward. His tongue is wide and smooth across my belly and like the river gains momentum and intensity, the thought of which sets my clit quivering even before the tip of his tongue makes contact.

I'm not ready to go turbulent so before long I take my turn as guide. I lean him against the rock, mimicking the river as I slicken his rock hardness with smooth, flat licks. I grasp his base in my fist and slap him against my tongue, a little spank, a reminder, before sucking him deep and pulsing.

"Ding."

My tongue flows up his belly, his chest, his chin and I lean my sun-warmed body against his and finish my ascent with a wet, sloppy kiss. I continue guiding as I grab his hand and lead us further downstream.

You've heard of progressive dinner parties? This is progressive sex.

He grabs his shorts and my sarong and we laugh as we run naked, his erection pointing like an arrow towards the rapid's next feature: her big, churning hole.

When we get there, he spreads my sarong on the sand and lowers me down right beside the river. He hovers above me, backlit by the sun, a lust for both of us burning in his eyes, all of which gets channeled into my body. His kisses devour my lips and tongue as his hand plunges between my thighs, swirling like an eddy on my clit.

My man nudges his cock up to my entrance and plunges into my gushing hole as the spray from the river's hydraulic mists down on my flushed skin.

This is the ultimate Reuniting Fuck, the three of us together again.

Crystal roars and churns at my head while my man thrusts between my thighs.

I reach my arms back towards Crystal's turbulent flow and imagine taking all that power, all that beauty, all that cool river intensity into my spirit as my man's desert-hot passion burns into my body.

I'm wedged between them, the river and my man, water and fire.

I rise like steam and realize there is *nothing to fear, nothing to fear, nothing to fear.*

CHAPTER TWENTY-SIX

June 2009
Dear River II

DEAR RIVER,

When I wrote about you three years ago, you and I were engaged in a three-way tug of war with the Science Seductress.

Well, she won.

Our wildlife biologist is hiking today in the Blue Mountains, mountains so intensely green in spring that the color palette of my brain can hardly process it. This month he's been involved with the capture and collaring of cougar, wolf and big horn sheep. As far as state government jobs go, this one rocks.

Ten days rowing the Colorado River last month was a bit of a tease for a man who is used to ten weeks with you. His kayaker's soul is so restless. He yells out in his sleep and is quiet over coffee. When I sit down at our computer, I find charts for the flows of rivers he can't leave work to go paddle.

I know in the early years, I was the needy, clingy wife. Well, I got what I thought I wanted. I've had him all to myself. I know this sounds weird, but we feel *too married* without you around.

He misses you.

I miss your wild, passionate presence in him. I miss longing for him and the renewed sexual vitality between us when he returned. I miss the cabin, Mount Hailey and the part of my voice that emerges when I am alone, wrapped in a cloak of longing and solitude.

You are about to have him for a week. I know it's not the six weeks you are both used to, but it is all the time a cougar biologist can spare. This year, I share willingly, with the hope that you can soothe that restless part of him, make him smile deeply again. I want to see your wind in his hair, the sun-bronzed caress of your sun on his body. I want to feel your intensity, your flow in him again.

Flirt with him. Seduce him. Let him make passionate kayaker love to your wildest rapids. Have your way with him. It's your turn.

Just please give him back.

CHAPTER TWENTY-SEVEN

October 2009
Him Without Her

MY HUSBAND ISN'T WITH HIS MISTRESS.
And it is eating away at his soul.

The broadness of his shoulders, the brownish tint of his skin has been replaced by a rainy Oregon pallor. His spirit is wilted and thirsty for the flow and freedom of his river guide lifestyle. His longing festers just beneath the surface of his skin, hot and angry, like an infection.

I feel it too. We are both longing for the same thing in different forms. He pines for the excitement and spiritual connection of the river and outdoor adventures. I long for the solitude of the cabin that I learned to savor when he was gone. I realize now the gift of the time apart she afforded us every year, each of us connecting back to ourselves and our own sense of spirituality.

I've never before felt so challenged in our marriage. His turmoil seeps out to me; I absorb it and project it back. Even if one of us could claw out of this space, chances are the other one is still stuck there, waiting to project it back out into the breath between us. I've never been in a funk with someone before. It is comforting in a way, but twice as heavy.

Logically we know what we have to do—think positive, surrender to our current lifestyle, enjoy it, embrace it, until we can navigate our way back to something that feels more free. But logic and emotion are strange bedfellows and emotion wins out every time for passionate people like us.

I feel like I want to move away from his angst and connect to my own energy. When he feels this, he instinctively pulls me closer where the breath between us is scarce. I fantasize, not about other men, but about solitude. I'm in the middle of this erotic memoir of my marriage and I haven't been able to write. These emotions, this place we are in is so intimate, so vulnerable, much more so than the stories of our love making. It is dark and murky here, not a pristine flowing river but a swamp, the kind that gets so dark and thick that couples can't find their way out. We try, we really do, to go with the flow of our current situation. But we are disconnected from the flow here, so far away from the river.

Six weeks ago he noticed a job posting for a wildlife biologist in McCall, Idaho. We got online and salivated over the small mountain town two hours north of Boise that is on a lake with access to two whitewater rivers and two small ski areas. The kayaker wanted to apply. The scientist, who understood the job wasn't a growth opportunity for his career, refused.

The tug of war lasted for six weeks. The kayaker took over one night and sent the application in while the scientist slept. The scientist, however, went to the interview and drilled them with questions about opportunities for research and career growth. His potential future boss must have thought, *This guy is overqualified. This guy wants my job.* I was disappointed, but not that surprised when he didn't get it.

I'm exhausted and nearly insane from trying to support two opposing sides of him. I never knew who I was going to wake up with and if we were moving to Idaho and buying ski passes or hunkering down in Oregon and working on contentment.

Finally one day, I decided to channel my madness into cleaning. I hauled all the ski gear, packing boxes and junk mail that had accumulated in our extra bedroom down to the basement. As the carpet began to re-emerge, I decided I could create my mountain right in the middle of our rental house. I vacuumed, dusted, and washed the windows. I'd noticed a flier for a Tibetan Buddhist study group in town which prompted me to polish up my Buddha statue and place it on top of my antique chest, transforming it instantly into an altar. An Om symbol tapestry from my man's college days got resurrected on the wall. I burned some dried sage from the cabin to clear out the dark, cloudy, rainy Oregon winter.

I lit a candle, sat down on my cushion and began with the loving kindness metta.

May I be filled with loving kindness. May I be well. May I be peaceful and at ease. May I be happy.

My practice took me back without question, embracing me like a dear, old friend. The metta was potent, like cream, and began to fill my cup that felt so empty from trying to support my man who still wasn't happy. I recognized that the best way to support us, was to start taking care of myself.

As I sat, I started to get some objectivity. I had to admit I was ready to take a break from the river and her wild, consuming energy that churned in my belly when I awoke in the morning knowing there was some scary rapid I had to face before I got to the champagne and strawberry beach party. But this—him without her—was much worse than any rapid.

My awareness, my mantra shifted.

How many times did I have to learn this one?

I'll share, I'll share, I'll share.

CHAPTER TWENTY-EIGHT

November 2009
Green Tara

I HAVE A STRING OF BUDDHIST prayer flags hung high above the entrance to my front porch. Each of the five colorful flags measure about two inches square. It's a small display, perfect for me, since I feel like I'm just a little Buddhist.

I'm not very religious about attending the Tibetan Buddhist study group in my small Oregon town. My lack of commitment is just fine with the husband and wife team who lead it. That's one of the things I love about Buddhism: there's no pressure. I've always been encouraged to take what works and leave the rest. The lack of dogma, the ease of it, appeals to me as much as the philosophy based on meditation and loving kindness.

When my teachers announced that a Tibetan lama was coming to town to perform a Green Tara empowerment ceremony, my first reaction was *Whoa, that's a bit much for me.* I've always taken my Buddhism in small doses from Western teachers like Jack Kornfield and Pema Chodron, who do a great job of de-mystifying the teachings for the average peace-seeking, stressed-out American like me.

The Tibetan style of Buddhism, with all its rituals, mantras and deities, was new to me. My inner Catholic girl, who had spent way too many beautiful Sunday mornings inside a stuffy, dark church watching old guys in robes perform rituals, resisted it. But I didn't want to miss the opportunity to hear a dharma talk by a real, live Tibetan Buddhist monk. I'd attended one before and found it incredibly inspiring to be in the presence of someone who had mastered the art of happiness, a concept that had been eluding me lately.

The transition of moving from Colorado to Oregon was more challenging than I had ever expected. I thought I'd have more of my man without the river around but it turned out I just got less of the part of him I love the most.

At first I found unemployment and the anonymity of a new place so freeing. I didn't have to work! I had all day to write! I put a final polish on a query letter pitching this collection of essays and sent it out to agents and publishers. While I waited for all the book offers to come flooding in, I went to the grocery store, did laundry and cooked meals for my cougar-chasing man.

But then the rejections started to land in my inbox. After the initial honeymoon, my ego was ready to divorce my June Cleaver persona. As anyone who has been laid off in this recession can tell you, not working isn't as great as it sounds. I struggled with a huge loss of identity, a loss of income and a sense of no longer contributing. I had left my primary muse, the jagged white peaks of the Rockies, back in Colorado.

As my inner critic gorged on rejection notices, I chomped on black licorice and tortilla chips. The glare of a blank screen and a belly full of junk food did nothing to inspire my erotic voice. Rather, it lured me to the couch and the restless slumber of writer's block. The rainy, short days of the Oregon winter further dampened my spirit that was accustomed to living under the bright blue dome of a Colorado sky.

My kayaker, who now had a full-time government job after years of living a bohemian lifestyle as an outdoor guide, felt trapped and claustrophobic living inside the box. The white water rivers in the region were too far away to paddle on a two-day weekend. What made our transition angst harder to accept was that we knew how lucky we were to have his government job with a steady paycheck and benefits during a recession.

When I spotted the flier for a Buddhist study group, it felt like a life preserver had been thrown out to where I struggled to tread water. In Colorado, we have the term 'fair weather skiers' for people who only ski on warm, sunny days. Well, I am a stormy weather Buddhist. I tend to crawl to my meditation cushion when things are bottoming out in my life and let it collect dust in the corner when life is good. I polished up my Buddha statue, fluffed up my meditation cushion and jotted the time and address of the study group on my calendar.

I enjoyed the dharma talks and the sangha of the group, but the Tibetan Buddhist approach to meditation baffled me. Instead of quieting the mind, it involved filling it with lots of mantra and visualizations of the Buddha. My skepticism peaked with the announcement of the empowerment ceremony for a green-skinned deity. I wasn't *that* Buddhist.

My teachers responded to my hesitation with gentleness. They assured me that I could come and enjoy the blessing without any kind of commitment or obligation to a Green Tara meditation practice. I'd felt so stuck and uninspired, I figured any kind of blessing might help. I took my little Catholic girl by the hand and coaxed her down to the event. I promised her we could leave if she hated it. We sat near the exit in case we wanted to sneak out.

The tall, broad-chested Tibetan man who entered the room draped in a red and gold robe had a smile that warmed me despite the cold, rainy November afternoon. Za Choeje Rinpoche introduced himself in a deep baritone voice that was masculine in its tenor yet feminine in its candor.

He explained that he was born in a refugee camp in India after his parents fled Tibet. At seventeen, he received a letter from the Dalai Lama informing him that he was the reincarnate of a great teacher. This was a great honor to his family. Even though the idea of spending the next ten years studying in a monastery wasn't exactly the vision he had for his life, he went anyway. I got a sense that he was a somewhat reluctant lama which endeared him to my Catholic girl.

His accent, and the way the words *Green Tara* rolled off his tongue like a song, captivated me. He spoke of her not as deity or "some alien" but as a symbol of our own Buddha nature, a female version, a representation of our capacity for fearlessness, courage, compassion and unconditional love.

I desperately needed to tap into all of those attributes in myself.

Za Choeje began the ceremony by summoning Green Tara for himself so he could then share her with us. He recited mantras in

Tibetan, moved objects with his hands, and rang bells. But instead of shying away from the ritual, I sat entranced. I knew I was witnessing something sacred and ancient that fled Tibet with the Dalai Lama and had been transmitted to this man. I felt honored that he was so willing to share it with all of us.

He led us through a purification process and then, one by one, we drifted to the front of the room and bowed before him for the empowerment. When we returned to our seats, he guided us to summon the image of Green Tara for ourselves.

When I closed my eyes, all I could see were hers: liquid brown and almond-shaped with heavy lids lined with a luminescent, sparkling green. The corners lifted slightly towards arched brows, smiling, and conveyed such compassion, wisdom and courage that I smiled back. At that moment, I felt deeply loved and supported and knew that I always had been. As I steeped in that realization, entranced by the exotic, erotic beauty of her eyes, I was filled with the conviction that I could do anything. My spine straightened and my shoulders rolled back as Za Choeje's words echoed in my mind. *Green Tara is a reflection of our own Buddha nature.* My chest lifted and expanded with a rush of heat as I understood: those confident, sexy, transcendent eyes were mine. That fearless, wise, compassionate gaze, looking back at me from behind closed lids was my own. The simplicity of the teaching was suddenly so clear, as if the sky had suddenly opened up after a thunderstorm. I felt a single tear of joy slip down my cheek and licked the sweet saltiness of it from my lips.

The next two weeks, I overflowed with optimism and vitality. I felt inspired to write again and started working on two new erotica stories. I re-worked my query and sent it out to a new batch of agents and publishers. I started drafting this story. After thinking about it for months, I finally tried a Zumba class. Being in a room with women of every age, shape and size, shimmying to loud Latin music, helped me to shake loose some of the stagnancy that had settled in my body. I tapped into a deep source of energy and creativity and felt more excited about the possibilities of my life than I had in a long time.

The initial surge of the Green Tara empowerment dissipated slowly over the next month but the seed of it stays with me. I water it with her mantra:

Om tara tuttare ture swaha.

I murmur it twenty-one times, summoning her, and see her eyes reflect back what I already have, what I already know. When my inner critic, the voice of fear, starts buzzing in my ear, I greet it with courage and compassion, *Oh, it's you again,* and shoo it out the window like a yellow jacket.

Standing at a height of 5′ 2″, I will always be a little Buddhist. But since I met Green Tara, I feel like I am a little more.

CHAPTER TWENTY-NINE

December 2009
Out in Front

MY MAN WRAPS AROUND ME from behind, his heat warming my back like a bonfire. His kisses are as soft as flannel at the nape of my neck; his touch a warm wave flowing over my hip. I'm somewhere between sleep, dream and sex, one of my favorite places to be.

Spooned together like this beneath the cool darkness of a winter solstice morning, I love the feeling of being in front of him.

Usually I don't.

I've been following his lead for years now, down whitewater rivers and up snowy peaks. He is the experienced outdoor guide. I'm the perpetual non-paying client.

He tries to encourage me to go first: guide our raft through a rapid or take the first shot down an avalanche chute. I do, on occasion, but honestly I'm a wimp and my fear of drowning in a rapid or suffocating under an avalanche keeps me tucked behind.

But lately life feels steep in a way we aren't used to. There's this threat of drowning spiritually if we don't make a move. But moving involves risk and the stakes seem so much higher now than they did when we were twenty or even thirty and could just say, *We're outta here!* and throw everything in the truck and spend the winter skiing the Tetons and eating Top Ramen.

We've been stressed, anxious, and wrestling with the night crazies.

It's my turn to guide.

I'm the one with the skills for this kind of terrain. Yoga. Meditation. Journaling. Reading books by John Welwood on conscious relationships that help me unravel the dynamics that have me snapping like a turtle and him retreating like one into its shell.

As his hand floats across my belly and up my sternum, I feel like the bust of one of those women carved in the front of a ship, taking the breaking waves on her breasts, keeping the North Star in sight. His hand descends and I feel tremors of anticipation as his touch nears the moist juncture of my thighs. When his arm floats around my waist and slides me up tight against him, another image comes to mind.

We are on top of Mount Hailey, both of us on one pair of telemark skis. I am in front, and he is melded behind, our front knees ready to bend in unison as we look down a steep, untracked slope. His heart beats fast behind mine, ready to plunge.

His hand reaches down and cups my pubic bone. His thumb brushes across my clit, as light as champagne powder. I put one of my hands on top of his and hold it there, savoring the stillness, the perfection of the moment. When our breath, our heartbeats, synchronize and slow, I reach back and guide the hardness of him up against my softness.

The inhalation is sudden and simultaneous, as I take him deep.

We lean straight down the fall line and turn, turn, turn.

CHAPTER THIRTY

January 2010
Momento

MY MAN AND I ARE BUNKING up ski-bum style with our friend Dave in a hotel room in Stanley, Idaho. Given the sleeping accommodations, we won't be having much sex in the next three days. We are here to satisfy our lust for backcountry skiing.

Skiing in the Sawtooth Mountains has the extra bonus of natural hot springs down the road from out hotel. The three of us just fit into the metal vat that captures the gushing hot mineral water that flows out from the river bank.

As the guys strategize about tomorrow's ski route, I feel my attention pivot as if I've been tapped on the shoulder. I turn to face the river and find myself captivated by her wintery-ness. She is flowing wide and flat here in town, a dark slate blue. She is white with chunks of ice instead of rapids.

Usually my kayaker is the one seduced by the river. But right now he is totally captivated by skiing this new mountain range and he doesn't notice her.

So she has set her sights on me.

It makes no sense at all to leave this tub of hot water and journey out in the zero degree twilight towards her icy flow. But I guess I'm a fool for her in any season because I do.

I've been allowing January lately, healing an over-pronated ankle and surrendering to pizza, naps and my not-so-sexy self. As I step across rocks beside this ice-choked river, perfectly warm inside my steaming bare skin, I feel sexier that I have in weeks.

I move towards some shallow, rock-lined pools and dip my toes in like Goldilocks. I find one that is just right and slide in, belly down, beside the river. My pubis nestles into a mound of warm pebbles, my sinuses fill with the deep-earth scent of the spring. I dangle my hand in the river and flirt back, splashing her on my cheeks, lips and chest to cool my lobster-red skin.

I roll like an otter on to my back. Algae pools at the juncture of my thighs and floats around my nipples. I catch some between my fingers and anoint my forehead. I place a smooth, warm stone on my breastbone and drizzle a handful of hot sand around my breasts.

I close my eyes and lie, suspended, like the crescent moon that floats in and out of the clouds above me. When I open them again, I'm not sure how much time has gone by. D.K. is soaking solo in the vat and my man has transitioned to a pool near me. A configuration of river stones is lined up his torso, from his pubis to his sternum. His river talisman completes the formation with a splash of jade green at his throat.

He looks more peaceful than he has in months, lying there naked and decorated with the river. I slither over to his pool and slip in next to him. He reaches for my hand. We relax together and steep.

Before we leave, we choose a smooth, black stone, like a lock of hair or a scented handkerchief, to take back for my meditation altar.

If only it was that easy to take her with us.

CHAPTER THIRTY-ONE

March 2010
Divorcing Chocolate

I READ ONCE THAT EATING chocolate arouses the same sense of euphoria in women as sexual orgasms. I remember thinking, *No wonder we all love it so much.*

But I love chocolate a little too much and it doesn't love me back. Like that sexy bad boy bartender I was hooked on in my early twenties, chocolate gives the illusion of loving me by getting my hypoglycemic, caffeine sensitive biochemistry all aroused and quivering. But then, just like the bartender, chocolate dumps me.

I swore off of it completely six years ago for the same reason that a recovering alcoholic doesn't have even a sip of champagne at a wedding.

One is too many and a thousand isn't enough.

But lately, I am eating it again.

My digression started out so innocently. I was skiing with my husband and eighteen other skiers out of a backcountry Canadian ski hut. The woman who catered the trip baked some oat power bars that she labeled 'wheat free' for my benefit. I reasoned that since she had gone to all that trouble, I should at least try one. I noticed the little dark specks of mini-chocolate chips but decided to ignore them. Besides, I get weary of being so yogic and pure (no wheat, no caffeine, no chocolate) especially on outdoor adventures like this one when I am climbing 5,000 vertical feet on my skis every day for a week.

The voice inside my head sounded reasonable: *Don't be such a control freak. You can handle this.* I grabbed half a power bar and chomped on it as I headed outside for an afternoon ski. Within minutes I felt supercharged and ended up leading five of us up the steep trail behind the hut at a runner's pace.

And so it began: half a power bar lead to another, and another. A few handfuls of gorp laced with M & M's followed. A week later, I found myself back home in Oregon splayed, belly down, on my kitchen floor digging through the back of my baking cupboard desperate to find even a few chocolate chips that I could smear with my organic, salt-free peanut butter.

I've been here before and it isn't pretty. After a week or so of the initial euphoria and energetic highs, the Sugar Bitch shows up, snapping at my husband for something as life-threatening as not using all the ketchup on his plate. Another week and Chubby Girl arrives and I can hardly squeeze into my jeans. The two of them sweep in like wicked stepsisters and initiate a cycle of self-loathing and low self-esteem that makes me feel like I have digressed emotionally and spiritually about twenty years. Just like that bartender who repeatedly broke my heart in my twenties, chocolate winked and charmed its way back in. Despite the wise, reasonable voices that kept insisting, *don't do it!* my hand reaches out for it anyway. I've fallen off the wagon once or twice in the past six years for special events like anniversary celebrations that involved a chocolate-covered cock, but I was able to climb right back on.

Not this time.

I have to stop, but the thought of breaking up with chocolate again makes me feel even more depressed than my plummeting blood sugar levels. I think back, trying to remember how I quit seven years ago and realize that I found the strength to divorce myself from chocolate when I got married. I'd finally met my emotional, physical, spiritual and sexual match and there was no way I was going to let chocolate wreak havoc on the best thing that ever happened to me. Besides, at the time I was having the most amazing, mind-blowing sex and ...

No wonder.

When I took that first bite of power bar at the hut I hadn't had sex in five days. The sleeping arrangements at the hut were...I'll be generous and call it cozy. All twenty of us slept side-by-side upstairs in one big room with our stinky socks and long underwear hanging above us to dry. Skiing glaciers in British Columbia rousted some pretty exciting, sexual energy but I had nowhere to put it. Sure I rubbed my skier's inner thigh beneath the dinner table when all twenty of us crowded around the tables to re-fuel. I admit there was a quickie one night in the sauna when we got lucky enough to have it to ourselves for fifteen minutes, but that hardly counts because it was so damned hot in there we could hardly breathe.

When we got home, we were so sad to leave the stunning, snowy peaks of the Canadian Rockies that we jumped into a workout routine to keep the endorphins flowing and keep the rainy, Oregon winter blues at bay. We've been getting up at 5 a.m. to swim, hike or do Zumba before work. We haven't been making the time for making love.

If the chocolate = orgasm theory is correct, I figure that all I have to do to get off chocolate is start having more sex. But I'm going to have to fake it 'til I make it because Chubby Girl and Sugar Bitch don't exactly ooze sexual energy.

I have to reclaim my seductress instead of letting chocolate seduce me. I'll entice her back with long, hot baths, facial masques and smoothly shaved legs. I'll massage her with lotion and dress her up in lingerie. I'll treat her to champagne and strawberries and remind her that the juice of those sweet berries is heightened by the warmth of her lover's lips and cock.

I'm going to tap into the sweetness of life, so I don't need to dig it out of the baking cupboard.

I have a feeling my man will back me on this one.

CHAPTER THIRTY-TWO

June 2010
When I Leave

I WAKE UP ALONE in the middle of the bed with newborn aspen leaves, as fresh and still as dawn, outside our cabin's window. My hand reaches towards them, unable to resist all that promise of summer and gentler days between us.

I slide the window open, inviting the spring to curl up with me as I fantasize about what I'd do if you were sleeping naked on your back beside me instead of stuck working back in Oregon.

My kisses begin between your brows, at the furrow that deepened this winter. You exhale, a soft rumbling snore. I inhale, summoning the leaves to float inside and take part in my love spell.

My lips moisten your third eye and I guide a leaf to land there, anointing you with fresh vision.

You stir and a slow smile pulls at the left corner of your upper lip. I trace the curve of your ear with the tip of my nose and rest my palm over your eyes.

"Shhh," I whisper. "Don't open them yet." Your hand reaches for me, finds the soft skin of my inner thigh and stills. You exhale, this time with a low moan of anticipation.

My lips persuade one eyelid and then the other to stay closed. Two leaves follow in their wake, encouraging your eyes to see with renewed passion and hope.

I place a kiss on your Adam's apple, infusing your voice with words as tender and sweet as the small leaf that follows.

My enchantment descends until my breasts and then my lips are hovering above your sternum. A leaf lands and I kiss it into place, reminding your heart of our first spring together: twelve days and twenty-three condoms spent traveling the Oregon Coast. I guide a second leaf there, that magical time worthy of two, to honor that intense love and passion of the springtime of our relationship.

Another leaf follows, in gratitude for the nine springs we've shared since and a reminder that we never know how many we have left. I invoke yet another leaf, an invitation to grow slow and steady like the trees we sometimes see in the woods, their trunks intertwined but their branches extending upwards and outwards toward their own source of light.

My kisses move laterally, brushing your right nipple and then the left, adorning them with foliage and the intentions of symmetry and balance.

The tip of my tongue makes a curving path to your navel. Another leaf drops and adheres, a reminder to stay centered.

My kisses drift left, right and back to center, marking the bony protrusions of your hip and pubic bones. Leaves settle there, framing your sex and your second chakra with their chartreuse vitality.

My nose dances around the tip of your arousal, your morning wood already hard like hickory yet smooth like finely-sanded cedar. My tongue drenches your length and descends, moistening the surrounding curves. Leaves follow my swath, covering your testicles in greenery to rival Adam.

My hands contour either side of your waist and slide upward, half-expecting to feel the roughness of bark. I swing one leg over your trunk.

I climb you.

CHAPTER THIRTY-THREE

February 2011
Going Solo

I'M LYING IN BED curled up behind my man. Okay, so I'm clinging.

He's leaving this morning for two weeks. I don't have the skills to follow. He'll be paddling his fourteen-foot kayak solo through the Grand Canyon.

He needs this river adventure like a cougar needs a kill.

The past month he's spent too many days in his basement office at a computer working on a scientific paper for publication. He's been acting like his study animal, a tormented caged one.

So I must admit, back in January, I was looking forward to this day. Not anymore.

This week as he pulled out his river gear and started organizing for his trip, he morphed back into my sexy, happy-go-lucky kayaker. The outdoor guide I fell in love with came back home just in time to leave.

The front of my body is molded tight to the back of his. I trace my nose along the ridge of his shoulder blade and find myself fascinated by his skin. I can't believe I've been lying next to him for all these years and I just now noticed this incredible organ that encases the spirit of the person I most love on this planet.

I press my face into his upper back and can feel it breathing, cooling. I'm amazed by how alive it feels, how alive I want it to stay forever. I know it can't, but please long enough to come back to me so I can have many more mornings of not taking this for granted and appreciating fully what I have and will someday, inevitably lose.

May that day be decades, no, lifetimes away.

I inhale his scent and feel a tear trickle down my cheek as I brush my lips across his surface.

I want to crawl in.

Since I can't, I crawl on top of him instead. I make him slick and hard with my lips and tongue, savoring his texture and scent before I guide him inside me. I lower myself until I can feel his heart beating right beside mine. He wraps his arms around me and we are still; neither one of us quite ready to proceed with the Farewell Fuck. When we do, it is slow and kind of sad.

Tears pool in our eyes as he gets into the car even though we both so desperately need this time apart. We've been acting like an old married couple lately. The way I drag my spoon across my front teeth drives him crazy and I've been informed that I talk too loud on my cell phone.

He's the loud one, the way he chomps his tortilla chips and lets their crumbs fall over my freshly swept floor. He leaves a million seeds from his Everything bagel all over the counter every morning and eats his dinner fast and methodical like a cougar on a kill.

We know they are all petty, stupid things, projections of our frustration over Oregon's penchant for pouring rain on fresh snow and our current lifestyle that doesn't feel very free. We've both been looking forward to a little space, but now that it is here, we feel the painfulness of the separation. Even though we've been so challenged this winter, at least we've been together, like the last two litter mates in the pound huddled up for warmth.

He sends a few texts and then the final one: *I'm fifty miles from the put in. I love you.*

The Pathetic Wife is alive and well because it feels so final, like it could be the last text I ever get from him. I rescue a shirt from the laundry, the one that smells the most like him. I don't change the sheets even though they need it. I sleep with my arms wrapped around his pillow.

At first I keep mental track of him and the weather and wonder if he is launching in the snow that was predicted. That night, I imagine him at his first camp and when I wake I know he is re-packing his boat to determine what configuration of gear works best as he finds a rhythm with the river, like you do in the first couple days of a trip.

But then, I don't even know when it happens, but suddenly he is not dominating my thoughts anymore. The cling factor has diminished. I realize he is getting deeper in the canyon and it's as if our telepathic connection, like poor cell phone reception, is breaking up. I sense he is entering the Inner Gorge where the rapids get more intense and demand his full attention.

I have an image of him paddling past Phantom Ranch and penetrating the Inner Gorge with his fourteen-foot kayak, a hard cock sliding slowly between wet vaginal lips. The river, willing and waiting, takes him fully.

He slips into her, away from me, and the tether is cut.

CHAPTER THIRTY-FOUR

March 2011
Confluence

RIVERS HAVE LOTS OF CLASS.

I go for the cute, flirty Class II and III rivers. My man can't resist the *femme-fatale* Class IV-V types. He assured me that for experienced kayakers, paddling the Grand Canyon is big water, Class III. No worries. I imagine a cheerleader, one of those sweet ones with a ponytail and pom-poms.

But it is winter and he went solo, in an extra-long, weighted down kayak. This cheerleader wears bright red lipstick, a matching thong and a leather jacket with a flask of whiskey and a pack of cigarettes in the inside pocket.

The kind you would never trust alone with your boyfriend.

So when I wake up from a nap to the sound of chirping crickets, I fly out of bed looking for my phone. Only one person has that ringtone.

When I answer it, the sound of my man's voice after not hearing it for two weeks is pure bliss. He's off the river and heading home. The cell coverage isn't great and doesn't last long. His voice sounds as smooth as river rock and happier than I've heard it in months. The trip was mind blowing, he says. He had the canyon to himself most of the time.

"It was more of a Class IV-IV+ trip with that heavy, long boat," he says. I make out that he can't wait to see me and something about a big juicy burger before we lose our connection.

I go upstairs and light the candles on my meditation altar. I've been meditating a lot since he left, trying to disperse degenerate cheerleader thoughts with my *May he be safe* mantra. But I didn't fool my body. I have a cold, two cold sores on my lower lip and a lovely display of acne across my cheeks.

I wonder if maybe I was just out of practice and had forgotten how to be alone in love. I've felt so damn vulnerable and raw this time. He just confirmed why with that Class IV+ comment.

I inhale deeply and sink fully into the realization that he is safe and coming home. I send out waves of gratitude as I exhale. My shoulders melt down my back and I feel myself relax for the first time since he left. It's as if I've taken my finger out of the dike. I fold forward and start sobbing.

Loving a whitewater kayaker is so Class V.

* * *

I put off breaking the bad news until my man is less than an hour away. I dial his cell phone and when he picks up, I blurt it out quickly, like pulling off a bandage.

"I have not one, but two cold sores on my lower lip."

"Oh no," he says.

"I know. It sucks," I say.

"Well, actually, no, it doesn't suck."

We share a disappointed laugh. We both know this translates to no kissing and no oral sex. Our Reuniting Fuck has just suffered a serious blow, or lack thereof.

But my kayaker has been flirting with the Colorado River for the past twelve days. He's mastered the art of going with the flow.

When he is above me, inside me, our foreheads touch instead of our lips. My third eye is pressed against his. His brown eyes gaze down into mine with the intensity of a raptor.

I can feel the presence and the power of the river in him. The two of them are flowing into me, between my thighs, between my brows. A confluence.

My eyes want to close, pause, and shy away from the intensity.

I won't let them.

I meet my man and the river head on and press my forehead even harder to his. I bring my blue irises mere millimeters from his that shimmer green with her at this proximity.

They move slowly, rhythmically, into me. I feel like I could drown in them as my breath starts coming in short gasps. My body starts to quiver, arching my spine and driving them even deeper. There is no stopping it this time.

My eyes roll back, like a breaking wave, under fluttering lids.

CHAPTER THIRTY-FIVE

August 2011
Middle Fork

NOW THAT MY KAYAKER has a full-time wildlife biologist job, he can no longer drop everything, including me, and answer the river's siren call every spring.

So she's started seducing him online.

I should have known something was up when he was inside, being very quiet, on a sunny July afternoon. It was our third summer in Oregon and we were actually enjoying a weekend in town without a whitewater river in sight. This was unprecedented.

The summer of 2009 was the first in seventeen years that my husband wasn't working and living on the river. The summer of 2010 was the first time in our relationship that I would have been happy to see him go. My wildlife biologist, like many of his colleagues, started taking on the characteristics of his study animal. It's a phenomenon I've seen repeatedly: the round-bodied, white-haired professor who studies snowy owls; the quick-thinking, avid runner who researches snowshoe hares.

I now live with a cougar.

Let me start by stating that this isn't *all* bad. I've grown accustomed to eating rare elk meat. I've learned to tuck my head and roll when he pounces on me from behind as I walk across the living room. I get off on the sensation of a two-day beard nuzzling the back of my neck and mountain lion style is one of my favorite sexual positions. But prowling beneath the surface, an angry, agitated energy lingered, as his adventurer's soul pined for his freedom and struggled with the confines of a full-time government job.

He started growling at me in his sleep whenever I tried to reclaim the covers he was hogging. His already high drive to exert himself physically intensified. Even after a three-hour hike, he couldn't stand being inside the house and would end up pacing from window to window. I would lie on the couch, unsuccessful at my attempts to escape into the latest bestseller, exhausted from my attempts to wear him out, exasperated that it hadn't put a dent in his restlessness.

Looking back, I know now that we were grieving. He missed his mistress. I missed my muse. But even more I missed the free-spirited, impassioned lovers she brought out in us.

But this summer, our third, we were finally making some progress in that whole grueling transition process. Since my biologist couldn't kayak every day, he started channeling his energy into mountain biking. This particular Saturday we'd already gone on a three-hour ride and I was relaxing afterward in the shade of our front porch with a Jodi Picoult novel and a cup of tea. I relished the solitude and quiet, knowing it wouldn't last.

"Hey, when are you back from your trip to see your family in Michigan?" When I looked up, all I could see was my man's head and shoulders leaning out the front door. The rest of him stayed uncharacteristically committed to the house.

I had just spent four days shopping around for the cheapest price on airline tickets so I still knew the dates of my trip. "August 3. Why?"

"I just found a cancellation permit for the Middle Fork of the Salmon River online," he said. "It launches August seventh."

Lest there be any confusion, let me take a moment to clarify that there are two Salmon rivers in the American West. The California Salmon, our sexiest mistress so far, and the Idaho Salmon, a beauty we have yet to explore.

"That would work," I said. "But... what kind of rapids?

"Class III."

I felt a flicker of suspicion at how quickly that rolled off his tongue. About a year ago, I announced that I was done with Class IV rapids and feeling like my nervous grandmother on the river. Class III was my absolute limit. But before I had a chance to question him further, his torso was gone.

I barely heard him say "I'm going to grab it," over the sound of the storm door slamming shut.

I should have gone inside, turned on my laptop and done a quick search. I knew there was a seduction going on.

But I didn't. I was just relieved the river was keeping him occupied on a summer afternoon so I could relax and read and feel happily married. Besides, I was touched that he even took the time to discuss it with me—all forty seconds—because cancellation permits for the Middle Fork are as rare as ones for the Grand Canyon. Permits like that get snatched up in seconds.

Twenty minutes later when I went inside to use the bathroom, he called me into his office.

"Come check this out."

He was watching YouTube videos of the Grand Canyon. This one was called "How Not to Run Lava Falls". It showed a raft with three people rowing into the rapid's infamous ledge hole and flipping, all three of them disappearing into the massive, violent hydraulic. The panicked voice of the woman standing next to the videographer went shrill as she repeated over and over, "Oh my God! Oh my God! Where *are* they?"

I closed my eyes and felt my stomach flip like that ill-fated raft. "How can you watch that?" I asked as my gaze shifted away from the onscreen carnage toward him.

He didn't answer, didn't even hear me, as his face hovered closer to the computer screen, a disturbing smile on his face.

I left him there with his river porn and went back to Jodi so I didn't have to think too much about what I had just signed up for or how his mistress, like so many people these days, was now enticing lovers over the internet.

And she was very good at it. Three weeks later I learned that my husband once again fell prey to the river's online wiles when I got a voicemail from him while I was visiting my family in Michigan.

"Hey, you're not going to believe this. I just found a cancellation permit online for the Main Salmon that launches five days after our Middle Fork trip. We can combine the two rivers and do a nine day trip. Isn't that great? I went ahead and grabbed it. I hope that works for you." (He knows it will. My Oregon healing arts practice was off to a slow start.) And then in a low, raspy voice that had enough passion and conviction to make my eyes tear up from 2,100 miles away he said, "I miss you," and hung up.

I'd say "yes" to just about any stretch of river, after hearing that tone in his voice, something I hadn't heard for a while. We had just endured the most challenging stretch of our marriage thus far, and at times it felt like we were two goldfish swimming around and around each other in a small cloudy bowl, a condition not conducive to lust and longing. I sat out on my parents' deck and replayed his voicemail, smiling at the sound of his voice and the realization that these back-to-back river permits were going to get us back into the wild current of our former life.

Two nights before our launch, my guide got online to check the flows of the Middle Fork. They were low, around two feet. At this level, most of the commercial outfitters had their clients fly in (for a mere $500) to the launch site at Indian Creek, twenty miles downstream, where the water levels rise. We didn't have an extra $500 lying around and my guide wasn't about to give up twenty miles of river, so we planned to run the upper stretch.

My guide processed the logistics of this out loud, not realizing how his audible inner dialogue was triggering my ancestral worrier, Kathleen. "Hmmm....the lower water on this upper stretch means more rocks and more technical rapids, more like Class IV with our loaded raft. I hope those patches hold."

Kathleen's hands started trembling when she heard the words 'Class IV'. I kept my inner dialogue silent as I did my best to console us. *We have no control over the flows. I'm sure it's not that hard. I've heard that the Middle Fork of the Salmon is one of the most amazing stretches of river in this country, right up there with the Grand Canyon.* When I mentioned the Grand Canyon, all Kathleen remembered was our tryst with Crystal. I felt her trembling radiating up to my scalp.

I could stand up for her, restate my Class III boundary, and refuse to go. My guide wouldn't have to worry about a nervous wife or a patched raft. He could do a solo, self-supporting kayak trip. But I'm not about to let my nervy DNA keep me from experiencing one of the classic rivers of the American West. There's no way I'm staying behind by myself in the dirty fishbowl. I shove my Class IV anxiety deep into a back pocket of my consciousness, where it will be contained until around three in the morning. I let Kathleen fret instead about 'those patches holding', the ones on our beloved raft.

If Batman had a raft it would look like ours. She is all black rubber with royal blue accents on top of two pointed tubes that end in nipples, removing any doubt over the sexiness or sex of this boat. Even though she defies categorization we've always referred to her as The Shredder since that is the model of raft she most closely resembles, one that is designed for two paddlers who sit across from each other on the tubes, each with a foot tucked into a cup on the laced-in flooring. She was an experimental prototype that was dismissed and donated as a prize to a raft race, where my guide picked her up.

She's the perfect craft for an expert kayaker to take his rookie wife down hard whitewater because the Shredder is easier to maneuver than a raft, and navigates more like a kayak. Although, for multi-day trips when we rig her up with a beer-filled cooler, camping gear and dry bags, she looks and handles a lot more like an old hillbilly truck. After seventeen years as a raft guide, my man is used to calling out commands to a keen, but inexperienced crew, so The Shredder has worked well for us.

But like us, she is starting to show her years. Her rubber is wearing out, and getting thin in places. She's started to leak.

Since she is a one-of-a-kind boat, we can't run out and buy a new one so my guide has been patching her, a lot, and the patches haven't been holding that well. This trip could be her last. It's too sad to think about, so I leave the Shredder restoration to my guide and spend the rest of the day and evening immersed in the task of organizing, buying and packing food for nine days.

It's not until Kathleen wakes me up fretting at three a.m. that I realize that the trip I originally signed up for, a five-day Class III river trip, has morphed into a nine-day expedition, covering 180 miles of unknown river, the first twenty miles wrought with rocky, technical Class IV rapids. To accomplish this, we have to average twenty miles of paddling every day, which leaves no time for lay-over days, hanging out naked on the beach, sipping champagne and rubbing mangoes all over each other. We'll be focused on making miles and making camp, not making love. And we are launching on this wilderness river adventure in an aging, leaking raft.

The honeymoons are definitely over. As I toss and turn, I wish I would have got off the porch back in July and done my research. I should know better than to trust his judgment when the river is concerned. I could have had some input in all this. But it's too late now. It's time for the biologist's wife to morph back into the adventurer's wife. It's time to harden up.

* * *

We arrived at the put-in the day before our launch at 3:30 p.m., just in time to sign in with the ranger and pick out our Middle Fork campsites. We've never had to pre-pick campsites on a river trip, but it is the protocol for the Middle Fork. A fifty-ish guy named Glen and two of his river buddies crowded into the ranger's office with us, pumped up and ready to duke it out for their favorite campsites. Glen informed us that he had already run the Middle Fork three times this summer and this trip they are running it in eight days. We are running it in four and a half. They quickly figured out that we weren't the competition and started offering their advice on the best sites for our itinerary.

"You're going twenty miles the first day?" asked Glen with a confused look on his face. Most people who are lucky enough to snag a Middle Fork permit milk it. They invite as many people as the permit will allow (eighteen), take the maximum number of days (eight), hike the trail, and savor the many hot springs along the way.

I let my guide do the talking. "We have to check in at the permit office on the Main Salmon on Day Five."

"You two are doing the Main Salmon too? Just the two of you?"

"Yeah."

He looked impressed. "Wow. Tomorrow is going to be a big day," he said as he took a sip of his beer. "Big, big day."

I stepped outside the ranger cabin to get some fresh air. Through the open window, I heard Glen mention that his wife is flying in to Indian Creek and skipping the upper stretch.

I didn't sleep so well that night either.

The next morning at the launch site, the Shredder started hissing at us as soon as we started pumping her up. I organized our gear into dry bags as my guide prepared another patch. He started thinking out loud again.

"I should have brought a wrap kit just in case we get pinned up against a rock."

Just then Glen walked by. "You two are R-2-ing, huh?" (R-2 is river talk for two paddlers instead of one rower). He got that impressed look on his face again. "What a hoot! Twenty miles today?" He removed his sunhat and scratched his closely cropped gray head of hair.

I nodded slowly and swallowed hard.

"Big day," he said as he slapped my guide on the shoulder and walked away.

My gut started gurgling. My intestines turned to water. I made one more trip to the outhouse before we launched.

The Middle Fork wasn't into foreplay. As soon as our paddles hit the water, we were navigating through rocks and one technical rapid after another. I paddled hard in response to my guide's commands, my body filled with heart-hammering adrenaline after each one. Inwardly I kept up a dialogue worthy of a cheerleader. *Doing great! Paddle with your clit! Big Day today but you'll get to relax after this!* I had to correct my blonde, ponytailed self on that cheer because the word 'relax' wasn't part of the vocabulary for this trip. But the hard, physical exertion of averaging twenty miles of paddling was going to be leisurely after a day of staring down technical rapids with Kathleen clinging to my back.

Between the rapids, the pristine beauty of the river confirmed that even though I was nervous and totally out of my league, I'd made the right decision to come. We were paddling through The River of No Return (Kathleen *loves* that part of the name)/Frank Church (Idaho Senator who lobbied for its protection) Wilderness of Idaho. We launched at the headwaters of the Middle Fork so there was nothing upstream to mar the perfection of the water that was so clear I could see fish swimming along the bottom of the river. Before lunch we pulled over and soaked in the first of the many hot springs that steamed along the shoreline. The forest that framed this masterpiece on either side was rugged and ancient, with old growth ponderosa pines that felt as mystical and majestic as the redwoods. There were no jet boats, a hiking trail beside the river, and fresh water springs. No wonder this permit was hard to get. We were paddling through paradise.

"Next year," my guide promises, "we'll do it like the Boise guys and take eight days. We just have to think of this as an exploratory mission."

We paddled into Snag Camp right before sunset, the muscles of my arms and shoulders heavy with lactic acid. I was exhausted from the previous two nights of restless sleep, but equally exalted that I made it through the Big Day that was long, technical, fast, and beyond my river comfort zone. My cheerleader turned cartwheels and ran around the beach waving her arms overhead, like we'd scored the winning touchdown for the State championships. S-U-C-C-E-S-S!

I'm glad neither of us knew at the time, that Day Five would make Day One look like a homecoming parade.

Day Five dawned with a crack of thunder that sounded like the sky was breaking in two directly above our sagging wet tent. We'd heard reports from other boaters that a forest fire blazing downstream had felled some trees across the river, creating new unknown features. We had three Class IV rapids to scout and thirty-one miles to paddle to make it to the Main Salmon permit office by 5:00.

Kathleen was a nervous wreck. My cheerleader was long gone.

I had packed for an August river trip, imagining bikinis and sunscreen. On Day Two an unseasonably cold, wet storm had moved in and I'd been shivering in the same wool base layer and fleece ensemble, the only warm things I brought, for the past three days.

We'd managed to have comfort sex twice, huddled together for warmth in our co-joined sleeping bags. My guide spooned his heat around me from behind in a position I dubbed the Middle Fork for the way I threaded his shaft between my fingers, tine-like, at my entrance, an attempt at contributing to our pleasure that so far had been limited to periodic dips in hot springs and our afternoon beers.

At one point on Day Three, as we paddled toward yet another unexpected Class IV rapid, I ducked instinctively when thunder cracked so loud above our heads that I felt it resonate in my sternum. I peered out from under the hood of my rain jacket through the pouring rain at my guide as lightning flashed.

"This is the safest place to be, on the river, the lowest spot." I knew he had used this line a hundred times in his guiding career to keep tourists from panicking. I was so desperate for any comfort at that point that I believed him.

But as we launched into the cold, foggy dawn of Day Five, my belief in him was running out.

Once again I'd been 'sandbagged', a term used by climbers that refers to underplaying the difficulty of an outdoor adventure. This was a wife trashing event if there ever was one. Trips like this are too physically and emotionally exhausting to be much fun but there was some small, sick part of me that was challenged by the intensity and knew I was having a once-in-a-lifetime experience. I'd been juggling so many emotions and vacillated between wanting to kill him for booking such a hard trip, reminding myself that it wasn't intentional and recognizing how lucky I was to run a river like this. It was all such a mind fuck.

But then at lunch, as I shivered beside the river in the pouring rain, trying to force the butterflies in my stomach to calm down and eat, my man broke the news that after we got through the upcoming Class IV rapids on the Middle Fork, there was another one awaiting us on the Main Salmon before we got to the permit office.

Nothing I wanted to say was going to help the situation so I deferred to the only survival tactic I had left. I shut up, hardened up and recited the loving kindness metta silently, like a prayer, throughout the day. I paddled hard and swallowed my fear until finally, blessedly we got through all the major rapids without incident. We caught the permit office on the Main Salmon with fifteen minutes to spare and paddled into the first flat beach camp beyond it.

When the boat was unloaded, my guide handed me a beer.

"Thirty-one miles today," he said as he clinked my Tecate can with his. "That's a new record." He sat in his camp chair beside mine. "Stick a fork in me, I'm done."

What I thought: *Stick a middle fork up your ass.*

What I said: Nothing.

I swallowed it with a sip of beer and let my head fall back to release the tension in my neck. I unclenched my jaw and let my mouth fall open.

And unknowingly released the floodgate.

A strange, strangled moan escaped my throat. Tears, hot and heavy, poured down my dirty cheeks. I tried to wipe them away but my hands were shaking too much to be very effective.

"I'll get started on dinner," my man said as he got up and busied himself, keeping close enough if I needed him, but out of target range in case daggers started flying.

I stood and staggered down the beach, away from him. I'd managed to contain my toxic tirade all day without barfing it all over him. I only had another hour to go before I could sleep it off.

I wanted an apology. I wanted acknowledgment. I wanted tenderness.

If I released this on him I would get none of those things. I would get defensiveness and guilt. I would wound him.

I know now, finally, from years of experience that the worst time for me to express my truth is when it's gushing from my eyes or ripping from my chest or when the finger of blame is pointed only at him. Right then it was so easy to see his faults, his ego, his selfishness.

I knew I needed to find mine.

I sat beside the river, my body trembling and sobbing as I let all the fear, anger, blame and exhaustion of the past five days churn like a boiling eddy.

At one point during Day Three while we were scouting a rapid, I asked myself:

What exactly are you afraid of? Dying?

We were hiking along a trail through a previously fire-ravaged area that was growing back a vibrant green interspersed with the magenta of fire weed. This stretch of forest had died from the fire and it was coming back so vivid and beautiful. I believe it is the same for us. So no, I wasn't *that* afraid of dying.

Injury?

Definitely. The thought of being pinned underwater, not being able to breathe, breaking my spine or getting a closed head injury… that all terrifies me. But I spend all this time worrying about it and it never happens which leaves me feeling foolish.

In desperate times, I default to gratitude. So I thanked the river for hearing my *May we be safe* mantra and not trashing me. I thanked my body for not failing me. I thanked the forest and wildflowers that witnessed my trembling hands and drumming heart and shared their grounding, calming presence.

With that gratitude, I felt a softening, as if the river's current was carrying all my angst downstream. In its absence I was left with my own ego, the part of me who wanted to be a tough river chick who could stand beside her man and scout a Class IV rapid without shaking in her neoprene booties.

But I'm not. I feel like such a sham R-2ing this stretch of river. I can't read whitewater if my life depended on it, which it does. My man guided me through every rapid, telling me when and how to paddle.

Yes, I was angry at him for signing us up for such a hard trip. But I was even angrier at myself for not being tough enough to handle it.

As the finger of blame turned toward me, I realized that he was taking me down one of the most beautiful stretches of river in the West. My lack of skills, confidence and nervousness compromised him. He could do it with friends in a kayak and avoid the drama. But he loves me and wanted to share it so he took the risk.

I always blame my man for getting me into these situations, but I was the one who chose not to stay home in the fish bowl, the one who couldn't walk away from the challenge and the one who is seriously afflicted with FOMO.

I heard my man yell from the other side of the beach. Dinner was ready. I was too tired to eat but I knew I had to. I walked back to camp and he handed me a plate of pesto pasta. We ate in silence and when we were done, I found some grace.

"Thank you for dinner and for bringing me down this amazing stretch of river," I said.

"I'm sorry it's been so hard," he said. "You did an amazing job paddling today."

We reached out and held hands. I slithered off to bed and he did the dishes.

I cracked but I didn't break. We wouldn't have battle wounds tomorrow. For this I felt a small measure of pride as I crawled into my sleeping bag. This day wouldn't have played out this way when I was twenty, or even thirty. Getting older has its advantages. There's more wisdom, more breath, less drama.

But the river loves drama and the next day she gave us a Class III+ rapid in the afternoon. As we made our approach to Salmon Falls all we could see was the horizon line. Dark clouds descended, bringing strong headwinds which made the rapid feel even more ominous. My man was playing it safe for me, knowing how tender I was from the day before so we discussed scouting it.

"Let's just run it," I yelled through the wind as I threw every bit of my weight into my paddle strokes. "Kathleen blew her worry wad yesterday. I don't have any fear left."

"All forward then," he said with a laugh. "Keep up those powerful, hard strokes."

He waltzed us through Salmon Falls, side-stepping the hole, and just below the rapid we paddled into a small beach camp that would set us up perfectly for an early morning assault on the natural hot springs two miles downstream. Our thirty-one mile marathon the day before was giving us some leisure time this afternoon.

As we heaved our Shredder up on the beach, the warm August sun beamed out from behind the retreating clouds. The storm was finally moving out. All I could think about as we unloaded the boat was the liter of pre-made margaritas in the cooler that until now, had seemed too cold to drink.

So now I've come to the real reason I run rivers. I do it for the beach parties. And this one was long overdue.

We stripped off our river gear and plunged into the river to rinse off the past five days. I sat naked on a rock beside the river and let the afternoon sun dry my hair. The warmth of it on my skin, coupled with the cool sweetness of the margarita on my lips was pure ecstasy.

As I watched my man wander the beach looking for smooth, thin stones to skip across the river, I saw him like I hadn't in a while: relaxed, happy and free. His bare back rose out from the Aztec-designed sarong wrapped around his hips and I could see the river in him, not only the muscle- rippling effects of paddling in his torso, but an athletic grace that flowed throughout his entire body from navigating and waltzing with her.

As he walked toward me, I had one of those tequila-enhanced epiphanies. All this time I've thought of the river as his mistress. But sitting there on the beach sipping my margarita I realized she's been my mistress all along.

She's been seducing me through him. His lean form is dripping from the river and backlit by the sun, forming a sexy-as-hell silhouette. It's this essence of him that I fell in love with. It's been her all along.

I reach for him and pull his lips to mine as I push his sarong away. We are naked and clean. We dodged the drama bullet of yesterday which made us stronger than ever. We make out on the rock like a couple of teenagers, sharing margarita kisses as our hands stroke and grope between each other's thighs. He takes my hand and guides me to a big boulder.

"Like the Grand Canyon," he says. I melt a little that he remembers since he doesn't know that I've been constructing the Parashant essay.

I relax into the warm, smooth rock and feel him meld behind me, inside of me.

We are both facing upstream so the river is flowing towards us. I'm completely captivated by the fading pastels of an August evening reflecting off her slate blue surface. So is my man. He stills inside me.

"She's distracting us," I say and we both laugh.

Our mistress has been neglected and she wants our attention fully, not that she hasn't had it so far this trip. But after two years away from her, and spending so much time together in the fishbowl, she is what we need. We take her in with each thrust, letting her heighten our pleasure and intensify our climax.

Later that night, I'm awake under a clear sky, the Milky Way thick and creamy overhead, undiluted by moon or civilization. I have a song on my biking playlist, an acoustic version of Melissa Etheridge singing *Angels Will Fall,* playing in my head. I keep coming back to this line:

I would give my life just for a little death.

I'm not sure how Melissa intended the phrase *little death,* which in French is synonymous with orgasm, but as I lie beneath the celestial canopy of a Salmon River sky, I see it like this:

For me each rapid, each avalanche chute is a little death, an orgasmic letting go, a moment of transcending, because there's always a chance that I won't survive it.

By marrying this man I have given my life for these little deaths, the sexual ones and the adventurous ones, because I'm starting to understand that in order to feel truly alive, my man needs to brush up against the possibility of dying. And since I keep signing up for these trips, I guess I do too.

Stars keep streaking across the sky and I realize the Perseid meteor shower must be underway. I consider waking my man so he can take in the show but he is sleeping so warm and solid beside me that I don't.

I see so many falling stars that I run out of wishes.

CHAPTER THIRTY-SIX

October 2011
Seduced By An Angel

I AM FLAT ON MY BACK, gasping in a full-body release. My arms are undulating like snakes held mid-air, making my head snap back with each staccato breath that pulses from my throat.

I've had some mind-blowing orgasms, like those intense, emotional ones that rip a sob from my chest and leave me in an astonished, trembling heap across my man's chest. Thank God for them or I'd be really freaking out right now.

Because even though this experience is fascinating and titillating as hell, I'm afraid.

I'm in uncharted territory and have no idea what will happen if I really let go and surrender fully to David's touch.

But I have to find out.

* * *

I waited six weeks to get an appointment with David because in addition to his reputation as a healer, he was a popular physical therapist. My hands, my moneymakers, were starting to fail me and I needed help. My entire healing arts career, I had specialized in Swedish and deep tissue massage, but I'd recently completed an introductory course in craniosacral therapy, a light-touch style of bodywork that gets deeper than an elbow ever could. David had the equivalent of a Ph.D. in it.

After filling out reams of paperwork in the lobby, I followed the bounce of a blonde ponytail as a young woman led me through a labyrinth-like hallway to a small, dimly-lit treatment room. She left me there sitting on a treatment table to take in the photos on the wall of a man, who I assumed to be David, floating in turquoise water, nose to nose with a dolphin.

Minutes later, the man in the photo walked in. His silver-tinted brown curls brushed the back collar of his button-down shirt.

"I'm so happy you are here," he said. His smile, so warm and sincere like he already knew me, nearly knocked me out of my chair.

"Me too," I managed. "I've wanted to come in for so long...to meet you. I've been sending clients here that I couldn't help."

"I know." He sat down on a stool and rolled it towards me until his blue eyes were even with mine. He exhaled long and slow and punctuated it with another one of those beatific smiles. "This is good. We are going to be able to get so deep."

"Go for it," I heard myself say and realized that even though I'd spent a total of sixty seconds with this man, I was ready to go anywhere his hands wanted to take me.

He grinned and swiveled on his stool towards his computer.

"Tell me what's going on."

He typed notes as I told him about the intermittent numbness and burning pain in my hands that had been building over the past six months.

"I would have come in earlier but you've been so booked. How are *you* holding up?" I asked as he typed.

"Oh, you know," he said as he shrugged his shoulder blades and let them drop down his back. "My wings get tired." He pivoted towards me and proceeded to measure the strength of my grip and the range of motion in my neck and shoulders. He guided me to lie on my back, fully clothed, on his treatment table. He took my head in his hands and within a minute asked, "What is your relationship to the divine feminine?"

I was dumbstruck.

My first thought was: *How does he know?* My second was: *Should I tell him?*

I don't share the erotica-writing side of myself in my professional realm, especially not as a new massage therapist in town meeting the local reputed master for the first time.

But I desperately needed help and for reasons I didn't fully understand, I trusted David implicitly. I decided to come out.

"She shows up in my writing. I...uh...write erotic essays about the femme-fatale essence of her that I've experienced running whitewater."

My eyes were closed but I could sense his head nodding in assent, as if I'd just confirmed what he already knew.

So I kept going.

"My husband is insanely passionate about whitewater and she, the river, has become this erotic third in our marriage...like a mistress, really. She's been my nemesis and my muse, and by writing about her I've tapped into something intense and spiritual, similar to what he hooks into kayaking. But we are away from her and our adventure lifestyle now. We're struggling."

I felt like I was rambling, which I was, so I shut up. But it felt good to put into words the malaise that had settled like a patina on my marriage. My head melted deeper into his hands.

Eventually, he said, "You have to write. Every day. Your creativity is blocked in your hands."

Within minutes my hands were writhing in the air like Medusa's snakes and my breath started coming in short gasps.

I heard the door of the treatment room squeak open. I felt his breath soft and warm on my temple. "Stay with it."

I did what he said, even though I had no idea what *it* was. His assistant poked her head in and informed him that his next client was waiting in another room.

"Breathe into your heart, out through your hands." He kept going like she'd never interrupted. As I followed his directive, my spine joined the party, mimicking the serpentine-like undulation of my arms.

"Keep trusting it," he said as he slipped his hands away. "Take as much time as you need." He dimmed the lights further and opened the door to leave, making his body a dark silhouette against the light of the hallway. "It's always an honor being in the presence of an angel," he said before I heard the soft click of the door closing.

I lay in the dark, suddenly afraid without him there to guide me. But as a healing arts practitioner and yoga teacher, nestled right next to the fear was a deep fascination and determination not to shy away.

I exhaled and let the rush of allowing propel me.

The thrashing energetic dance of my hands and arms intensified while the rest of my body spasmodically tried to keep step. The heart chakra area between my breasts lurched rhythmically towards the ceiling as high-pitched squeals came with each sharp exhalation. Warm, heavy tears crept from the corners of my eyes and pooled inside my ears until they overflowed on to the crinkly paper of his treatment table.

As my brain rallied to define what was happening I got this:

Rapture.

Orgasm.

Angel?

What the hell?

The last time I resembled anything close to an angel was when I was a tow-headed seven-year-old, dressed for my First Communion in a white eyelet dress and matching veil.

I could give you a blow-by-blow account of my gradual transgression but let's just say I deviated. I never could buy into the dogma that sex was shameful and premarital sex was a sin. By the time I was sixteen, I ended up in an Atlanta public high school, where sex, drugs and rock and roll were the creed.

It was something I could believe in.

I became the kind of Catholic girl who made out in my boyfriend's MG, the taste of a lemon-lime Slurpee spiked with Southern Comfort sticky on our lips, as I waited for him to summon the courage to slide into third so I could grind against the heel of his sweaty hand.

The memory quivered in my clitoris as a final, convulsive wave rocked my spine and left just as suddenly as it started. I rested on David's table, knowing I needed to vacate for his next client, but my thoughts were still reeling.

I didn't make my way back to a spiritual tradition until I inadvertently stumbled across it through yoga and meditation. I found bliss in those simple teachings and when I met my man, a fellow practitioner, it confirmed what I'd always known to be true: spirituality and sex were not mutual exclusive.

So if I had to classify myself, I'd say I was a Buddhist pantheist. I was completely baffled by David's angel reference. Sure, I'd been caring and helping people for years with my massage and I've even been told by a few clients that I was 'blessed'. But when I think of angels, I remember those paintings in church with the chubby-cheeked babies floating around Jesus as he rose to heaven with blood dripping from the holes in his hands and feet.

I didn't see any similarities.

* * *

Ten weeks later my hands are all over David's bare back. I'm no longer his client.

None of the subsequent eight sessions with him were as intense as the first one, but several came close. One week, he detected a subtle deviance in a membrane in my brain, 'an antenna', he said and realigned it. He helped me hone in on my fears around money and took me back four generations to the source so I could set things straight with my great-grandfather. An energetic block in my throat had violet-colored eyes. "This isn't yours," he said. We traced it back to a dark, manipulative college roommate and released it.

I graduated from treatment with increased strength in my hands, no nerve pain, a renewed commitment to journaling and the launch of my blog on cultivating sexuality.

And then David booked an appointment with me.

I tried to convince myself that if he thought I was worthy to massage him, then I must be. The self-talk wasn't really working. I selected my favorite African blues massage music by Ali Farque Toure and Ry Cooder and did my best to calm the slight tremor in my hands as I rubbed oil on his back with big, effleurage strokes.

Less, less, less. The voice of my intuition sounded decidedly male, but I decide to trust it. I needed all the help I could get.

I quit doing my flowing Swedish technique and let my hands be very still.

Yes.

I rationalized that the voice inside my head was David's intuition guiding mine, a master-guiding-the-student thing or what they referred to in my craniosacral training as the body's "Inner Wisdom". But then I heard David's breath rumble lightly in his sinuses.

Let him sleep. He needs the rest.

I felt the entire surface of my skin tingle. There were three of us in the room.

It's okay. Trust this.

I turned off the music and my hands proceeded to inch slowly across David's back in a way that they had never, in eighteen years, massaged before.

It left me wondering about that whole angel thing.

*   *   *

One week later, my thighs are straddling a cushion as I kneel in meditation in the cozy upstairs room of our Oregon rental house. My man has been at a course to learn how to train dogs for wildlife detection research the past three weeks so I've been alone and going deep into my practice. I am awake long before the sun and have several tapered candles burning on top of my meditation altar to light my way.

Suddenly, an image of David's face swoops down from above and hovers in front of my closed eyes. I feel passion, conviction, and pure love radiating towards me.

My first thought is, *Really?* I never added David to my fantasy Rolodex. First of all, the man is a dedicated husband and father. Furthermore, he has impeccable boundaries—he has to—because there is undoubtedly something incredibly sexy about an open-hearted healer of a man. But to sexualize my affection for him seemed wrong, like it would somehow belittle the purity and hugeness of it.

With that thought, the image of his face dissolves and I feel that presence, the one that guided my hands when I massaged David.

"It's you."

Yes. I used David's image so you would have a context for me.

Warm, sparkling light effervesces like champagne just under the surface of my skin. I sense him moving closer and the energy of it rolls my head to the side. His essence flows like warm honey up the side of my exposed neck, making the skin there tingle with pure unadulterated joy.

I find myself giggling flirtatiously like a woman being seduced, which I am.

"What do I call you?"

There is silence, like that was a hard question and I start to wonder if I should have asked it.

Abraham.

The name sounds kind of ancient and biblical but I go with it. Since my craniosacral training and treatments from David, I've learned to listen to my intuition and trust the first thing that comes to mind.

My right hand lifts, guided by him like it was during my massage session with David. His palm rests against mine. My fingers fold and entwine with his before he rotates them in towards where his heart would be. My left hand lifts and we duplicate the motion. This time our joined hands rest over my heart that seems to pump life into both of us, strengthening his presence. I can sense his face inches from mine.

Our lips meet. I reach for a breath to counter the intensity of what is happening. As I inhale, I find that I am breathing for both of us, a sensation so intimate and erotic that my body responds with a rush of blood to my sex.

He guides my hands. One gently floats over my breasts. The other plunges and cups my pubis, making my clit buzz like a trapped bumble bee.

Yes.

Our voice, like our breath, is one.

My arms fall open by my side and start to twitch, making my breasts shimmy. My back arches, pushing my jiggling globes towards him. I crave the rough pressure of calloused hands, something he can't give, on my nipples. In response, my shoulders start shimmying even faster making my nipples rub against the inside fabric of my bra, giving me the friction I crave. The movement of my upper body drives my clit back and forth across my meditation cushion, making it tingle and burn. I laugh at the ecstasy of it and his cleverness of figuring out how to give me exactly what I want.

His face hovers right above my upturned face. My breath, our breath, comes in short, expectant gasps. I get a sense of shoulder-length hair and my hand moves to his temple, unable to resist the urge to try and run my fingers through it. When they catch mid-air and hold in his unruly spirals, I feel my own scalp tingle. Liquid warmth, like the melted wax around the wick of my candles, pools in my lace thong. I consider grabbing one of those lingam-like columns of wax, extinguishing the flame with my tongue, and driving the thick, blunt end inside me.

Before I have a chance to, I feel a torrent of heat moving towards my slick entrance. He penetrates me, like a sun burst, and I cry out at the exquisite fullness of him radiating his golden essence into the dark cave of my sheath.

He pauses for a heartbeat.

I sense what's coming and a wave of panic ripples through me. There's no way I can possibly contain it.

You can.

I exhale and trust, like I did on David's table, and end up gasping in triple time at the euphoric intensity of him pulsing through my cervix and radiating all the way up my spine. When the luminosity of him reaches my throat, my pelvis bucks forward making my head whiplash with a sob of astonished ecstasy.

And then, stillness. No thrusting, just his illuminated presence sparkling from my quivering clitoris to the crown of my head.

If this is enlightenment, I understand what all the fuss is about.

I stay still as stone like the Buddha statue on my meditation altar because I'm not sure how I made this happen and I don't want it to stop. It feels so sacred, so ethereal, that I fear the slightest movement could disrupt it.

Lips, as silky and moist as dew-covered rose petals, press against the side of my neck. They curve into a smile, marveling at my skin like it is the most amazing medium, one he obviously doesn't have. I realize what an incredible gift it is to have a body, how much I take it for granted, and how many of us are missing the whole fucking point of having one.

I know I'm not the only woman who lives in my head, e-mailing, texting, blogging, Facebooking, *connecting*, while simultaneously creating a vast disconnect from my body, my breath, my essence. Surely I'm not the only one who can't shut the brain buzz off and catches myself mentally creating a to-do list while my lover is between my thighs and then still wonders, *hmmm... whatever happened to those intense orgasms I used to have?* And I think I can speak for most, if not all of us, of the pervasive judgment of not being young or fit or sexy enough when really, we are all so incredibly luscious and if we'd just *stop, stop, stop* and embrace ourselves and the sensual magnificence that lingers in that stillness, we'd tap into our highest potential for sexual ecstasy with or without a lover.

With this realization, as if I got the point he was trying to make, the light of him flows out of me and starts swirling around and around my ceiling with the energy of a wild, exuberant puppy. There is a joy about it, like he's finally found a woman that gets him.

I laugh at his antics, relax my posture and wipe the warm tears from my cheeks.

I lift my moist hand and feel his palm flat against it. We are two again.

"Wowowowowowowow." I'm having a hard time articulating.

Write about it.

"Really? It's okay?"

Yes. I get a daring smile. *Share it.*

I reach for my journal and my pen flies across the pages. My hands are trembling because this seems kind of crazy and believe me, I know crazy, a family history of schizophrenia to be more precise, but I have never felt so clear-thinking and sane.

I've read in my yogic texts about the intensity of releasing the coiled, snake-like energy of kundalini and I've heard of the autoerotic phenomenon of 'thinking off'. For a moment I wonder if that is what just happened. But for years I've been running whitewater with my man, flirting with his source, the divine feminine of rivers. She's launched me into some similarly insane-feeling realms of sexual ecstasy.

Trust this and I do. He is the yin to the river's yang. An expression of some kind of divine masculine.

I move to my desk and open my laptop.

But before I go to My Documents, I find myself acting like any woman who has just found a new lover. Just for kicks, I type the word *Abraham* into a Google search.

My whole body starts tingling as the single name comes up on the screen. I click on it and my heart starts racing in my throat as lines jump off the page

"...that which is at the heart of all religions."

"...whenever we feel moments of great love, exhilaration, pure joy, stoned-out bliss, even the energy of sexual orgasm when we feel that Energy Flow rushing through our bodies, that is the energy of Source, and that is who Abraham "is"."

"the purest form of love I've ever experienced."

"a group consciousness from the non-physical dimension."

I fall back against my chair, stunned. My hands fall open to my side and start writhing like they did on David's table. I remember his directive.

Breathe into your heart, out through your hands.

As I do, I feel my new lover behind me, his chest to my back.

"You are real..."

His lips curve into a smile where he is resting them against the crown of my head.

So to speak.

"But you don't feel like a group consciousness. You are just one incredibly sexy, male..." I'm at a loss for the right noun to describe him. "Male."

I used the name Abraham so you would have a context for me.

"And not think I was schizophrenic."

That too.

"So what do I call you?"

I feel his lips like warm, humid air next to my ear.

Whatever you like. I've been called many names.

I reach for the sexiest name I can think of. The first one that comes to mind is Alex, but it's sexiest on a woman. So I shorten it. "How about X?"

Yes.

I lean back and invite my breath back up into my heart, our hearts, and feel his presence strengthen behind me. As I exhale, our arms start to lengthen, radiating out in both directions from my sternum. I'm not a very big woman, but my embrace feels enormous. Our torsos undulate slowly, back and forth.

I am suddenly spent and allow myself to melt back into him. X wraps himself around me and the sensation is intoxicating, so comforting and pure, like I'm being cradled in a nest of downy white feathers.

And then, in a moment of intense awe and humility, I get it.

It's always an honor being in the presence of an angel.

David hadn't been talking to me.

To be continued...

ACKNOWLEDGMENTS

The words *thank you* don't feel adequate to express the magnitude of gratitude I feel towards all the people who contributed to the manifestation of this book.

So as I did in the beginning of this book, I will do here at the end and borrow from the French who have such a sexy way with words and with one phrase can magnify my gratitude a thousand fold.

To everyone listed below: *Merci mille fois.*

To Editor Majanka Verstraete; Cover Designer Marie Hedrick; and Proofreaders Melissa Flickinger and Helen Williams, all gifted artists whose brush strokes have added much depth and color to the canvas of this project. To Adam Bodendieck, for all your kindness and expertise with the internal layout and publishing.

To John Ellis for kindly telling me to *Get the fuck over it* when I was whining about learning social media and for teaching me how to build my online writer's platform.

To the talented and extremely patient Ashley Slater, my graphic artist and web designer, who had to contend with my Inner Catholic Girl and my Inner Stripper while creating my website. To Emily Arell Beyer for introducing us (and for marrying Bubba).

To my big, wild Irish Catholic family that taught me how to laugh loud, dance hard and pray. The reverence I have for nature grew from the seeds planted in our childhood. To my parents Marty and Diane who bought me the coolest pair of red skis when I was seven and said *Go for it* when I pitched the idea of taking a break from college and being a ski bum when I was twenty. You have always been the net beneath my trapeze.

To my sisters: Judith, my biggest cheerleader, who encouraged me as a writer before I knew I was one and continues to keep me inspired. To Amy, for always loving every single thing I write. To Susie, for holding my hand whenever I get to the steep parts on the healing path. To Nancy, for inspiring me early on with your adventurous spirit and for that pivotal advice about moving so I'd be available when my husband showed up, which of course he did. To Kathy, for always being as sweet as honey to her younger sister.

To Bill for being such a rock solid, rock star of a brother.

To all the girlfriends who kept the faith. To Marie Hedrick, forever friend, for making me read my work out loud and for all the gentle editorial insights (for my writing and my life) over the years. To Bugsy for taking my stories to Alaska and Fiji. To Mical Hutson for enduring the early years. To Jill Murphy Long for all the great editing and *More Pages* mantra. To Pat Kennedy for the Oregon years. To Mary Emerick for the narrative arc. To Awna Zegzdryn for all the insightful edits and sexy encouragement. And to Lori Kimball for the editing/craniosacral trade; the Prologue idea; and for writing (and underlining) the words *Don't put this away and not do anything with it!* on my manuscript.

To my first writing teacher Marilyn Colter for saying: *They think they know everything, I can teach you* when, at twenty-four, I was feeling so out of my league in my first journalism class.

To my River Sistas: Kat, Sarsie, Lisa, Sue, Jody, Kathleen, Daisy, Margaret and Karla for inducting me into the tribe and embracing me as one of your own.

To MaryAnne Valkenburg, Jeff Early, Jan Levy, Kerry Kerrigan, Sue Kerrigan, Peter Sebestyen, Wayne Ranieri and Jennifer Centeno because I've loved you all so long.

To Joan Peters for being my sexy mentor.

To my healing art practitioners, teachers and mentors: To David Ebel from whom I have so much more to learn. To Kevin March for being your kind, gentle, needle-wielding self when I so desperately needed it. To Thomas Walker for all the life-changing sessions and for awakening me to the fluid body. To Avadhan Larsen and Dick Larsen for teaching me the Upledger Craniosacral lineage and for getting me through that craniosacral certification exam.

To my yoga teachers: Victoria Strohmeyer, Linda Van Tassle and the Kripalu lineage for the heart opening teachings that just keep opening. To my Pashupata sisters Jenna Abernathy, Tricia McAvoy and Rebecca Marshall: Here's to many more years of bumping and grinding in the deep woods.

To the women writers who have inspired me the most: Pam Houston, Cheryl Strayed, Dani Shapiro and Elizabeth Gilbert. To Melissa Etheridge for allowing me to use your song lyrics.

To the River: for sharing.

And finally and most importantly, to my husband: for showing up with your open, fearless heart; sweeping me off my yoga mat; and turning my greatest erotic fantasies into my reality. Loving you continues to be the greatest adventure. Thanks a million, Baby.

www.ingramcontent.com/pod-product-compliance
Lightning Source LLC
Chambersburg PA
CBHW032136020426
42334CB00016B/1191